THE HCQ DEBATE:

What Did Researchers Hide About Hydroxychloroquine?

Caxton Opere, MD

THE HCQ DEBATE!

What Did Researchers Hide About Hydroxychloroquine?

ISBN: 978-1-952642-04-3

To order additional copies, please call 469-459-1583.

Disclaimer
The information in this book is intended to inform healthcare professionals on a pandemic that has affected millions around the world. By reading this book, you agree not to hold the author or publisher liable for any information in the book. The author disclaims any liability, injury, loss or damage incurred as a direct or indirect consequence, of the use and application of any of the contents of this book. The books is sold without any warranties of any kind, expressed or implied. You agree that you and not the author or copyright holder, is responsible for any and all treatment or patient management decisions you make. It is your responsibility to check and confirm any treatments and dosages on any off-label use of drugs. The author does not guarantee that any website, url, government website, or links in the book will be functional at the time the reader purchases this book. Off–label and FDA authorized drugs may be mentioned and the healthcare professional should use sound clinical judgment in individualizing care to each patient. The accuracy of this work cannot be guaranteed and the contents of this book are to be used only as a guide and not as a substitute for sound clinical judgment, training, experience or a replacement for current treatment guidelines or consultation with an expert in the particular disease. All characters are fictitious.

Table of Contents

The HCQ Debate, Caxton Opere, MD

Introduction

Why are doctors fighting over the efficacy of hydroxychloroquine? Hydroxychloroquine (HCQ) is the α-hydroxylated metabolite of chloroquine used in the treatment of rheumatologic disorders such as lupus and rheumatoid arthritis as well as infections such as malaria. It has been in use for more than six decades with an established safety profile. When used carefully, patients can be on the drug for decades without much by way of side effects. HCQ has a higher tolerability and less toxicity than chloroquine. All of a sudden during the Covid-19 pandemic, HCQ suddenly became the "worst" drug on the planet, at least to some. If HCQ were a human being, it would probably have committed suicide. The amount of attacks launched on HCQ while seemingly politically motivated, seem to have far more than politics driving the discussions. A raging battle is going on between the scientists that don't care for patients and the medical practitioners that do prescribe the drug for their sick Covid-19 patients. The former are looking at data while the latter are looking at their patient outcomes. The scientists want to tell you how things ought to be done, the later are showing you the results they are getting using an inexpensive FDA-approved drug. By doing so those doctors prescribing HCQ are kicking the fear of Covid-19 in its teeth. While practitioners are not disproving scientists, scientists are bent on proving the practitioners are wrong for prescribing a drug that is helping their patients, despite the proof of improved patient care and reduced deaths. The stakes are rising each day, and what should have been a friendly banter on differences of opinion, has moved from a gentleman's debate into a caged ring fight, a bloody fight to the end. Doctors like Simone Gold are getting fired from their jobs for saying HCQ works. To be vilified for demonstrating that a drug as cheap as hydroxychloroquine works means there has to be something or someone behind the scenes instigating these attacks on practicing physicians. But the stakes are much higher than you actually think.

Two factions, scientists and practicing physicians, have narrowed their fight to just one thing, methodology. Rather than settle their differences amicably, and save as many lives as possible during this pandemic, scientists and practitioners have instead become bitter foes, locked up in an unforgiving contest where the winner takes all and determines the fate of the rest of the seven billion people on the planet. What should

4

have been an easy, friendly, logical scientific banter about the effectiveness of HCQ has been anything but friendly. So strange is this phenomenon of opposition between both parties, those vouching for HCQ's effectiveness in Covid-19 and those against it, that friends have stopped talking to each other based on how one feels about the use of the drug. On one side are research scientists, pharmaceutical companies and leading academic physicians backed by a well-heeled war chest of cash to spend, the power of the media propaganda machines behind them, and the backing of several high-ranking US government officials and institutions. On the other side are actively practicing physicians that have successfully treated sick Covid-19 patients. While actively practicing physicians continue to build an ever-increasing pool of Covid-19 patients successfully treated with HCQ either alone or in combination with other drugs, research scientists seem to be bent on disproving this reality. While patients are trying to share their HCQ success stories with the rest of the world, the media continues to shut them down while vilifying practicing physicians treating patients with HCQ or recommending its use for Covid-19 patients. When Michigan State Representative for the Democratic Party Karen Whitsett held a press briefing about how HCQ saved her life following Covid-19 infection, the Democrats launched an assault to discredit her; she had to file a lawsuit against her own Democratic Party assailants according to the *Detroit News*. On August 9, 2020, eight weeks after the Food and Drug Administration (FDA) had revoked its Emergency Use Authorization (EUA) for HCQ in Covid-19 infection, The *Washington Times* posted that New York City Democrat Councilman Paul Vallone, attested to HCQ saving his life. So far, no one has attacked the Councilman. So why would anyone not want patients to get a drug that seems to be helping patients with an infection that's already killed hundreds of thousands? Are those attacking the doctors prescribing HCQ even human, or are they just narcissistic robots bent on methodological inflexibility that could endanger the lives of millions? Or are they really interested in protecting sick patients from fraudulent doctors making false claims about a drug that lacks efficacy? Do they really care about the sick Covid-19 patients? They obviously have some concerns but are these concerns genuinely for the patient's benefit? If the drug works only for some and there is no other cure, why shouldn't those it works for get HCQ? Scientists claim there is no data to confirm what treating physicians are affirming. The doctors and their patients disagree with the scientists. Scientists have also claimed that they have designed clinical trials and that they have data to show that HCQ is not only ineffective in Covid-19, it is actually dangerous! And the beat goes on! So who is

5

The HCQ Debate, Caxton Opere, MD

right? That's the debate. Whenever such a controversy like this exists, each party is trying to protect or promote something. This book will provide facts to help you decide what each side may be trying to protect or promote. In the words of Lyman Beecher,

No great advance has ever been made in science, politics, or religion, without controversy.

The world is watching. Somehow, whether intuitively or because you already figured out the truth, even without having any medical training, you know that something is not right. This book is going to help you understanding that "something". While doctors in America do not agree on HCQ's efficacy, the scientific data supports the scientists, and the clinically relevant data supports the medical practitioners! In this book, you're going to take a deep dive into the world of scientific data in a very simple way that will help you understand the HCQ clinical trials from around the world. Even if you're not a trained healthcare professional or you are but just not adept at analyzing clinical trials, you should be able to see at least one reason why both factions are fighting, even if it's a bad one, and what you need to do about your patients.

Most practicing doctors do not enjoy sitting down to examine how a clinical trial was designed and executed. We just want to read the author's conclusion in the abstract section of the published journal article, even if the conclusion is wrong. So if you don't enjoy looking at published medical journal in details, you're not alone. It's like performing an autopsy. As a resident I used to wonder why we needed to dissect journals like a corpse. Until I realized how misleading some journals actually were on important clinical conditions such as we now have with Covid-19. With all the information available, I really don't know why both factions still disagree after examining all the relevant scientific data, particularly the research scientists who seem to pride themselves on their uncanny ability to analyze data. Those outside the United States, with the exception of some UK professors to be mentioned later, have figured out what to do about their Covid-19 outpatient treatment and don't bother themselves with the HCQ controversies. The patients can get HCQ over the counter. They go to the store, buy the HCQ, take it and get better without ever been part of the statistic or controversy. The patients who take HCQ, the doctors that know HCQ works for their patients and for them and their staff in the United States, are the ones in the line of fire. Hopefully, that would not be for long. Unfortunately at this point, those who are supposed to be arbitrators of both sides have turned and it seems they are traitors of humanity. These are research scientists and medical doctors conducting clinical trials, that don't seem to care about the human condition or the needs peculiar to each individual affected by Covid-19. While those against the drug cite research articles in reputable journal results vilifying HCQ, those with far above average skills dissecting these research papers often find they are inadequate to make the assertions they are making about HCQ's ineffectiveness or even worse, toxicity. Some of these papers have led to unnecessary but nevertheless drastic decisions affecting millions. For example, in May 2020, France banned the use of HCQ in Covid-19 patients following the WHO's cessation of its HCQ clinical trials which was in turn based on a Lancet May 22, 2020 paper that was retracted as its "data' could not be verified. We will look at some of these studies in this book and the similar conclusions they have made. You will be the judge on the value of these studies.

One question that has baffled many regarding the HCQ debate is, WHO IS RIGHT? Are the doctors claiming HCQ works right? Or are those saying it is ineffective right? Could they both be right or could they both be wrong? At this point in time, it would take an unbiased truly logical, investigative, scientific mind to answer this question of who is right. Or is all the debate just a mistake in communication? Perhaps the right question to ask is what is right, meaning, what is right for our patients? Should I prescribe a drug that a pilot study in France has shown to be effective in treating a condition that may be potentially lethal if left untreated or should I just fold my arms and wait for evidence? What will be the cost of waiting and is waiting a good strategy if death or hospitalization risks are the other likely outcome? Is there any real evidence to help a doctor decide on treatment and is it scientific evidence? What is the evidence for or against, the use of HCQ in Covid-19? How was this evidence gathered? Or is there something or someone more powerful, an agenda or a puppet master lurking behind the scenes, enjoying the conflict, that is driving the debate that has graduated to a life or death duel in the medical world of life and death? Does this HCQ debate or the entire pandemic itself have a historical replica that we can all draw from? Was such a history ever documented well enough to provide us with a template to draw wisdom from and avoid making the same retributive mistakes that befell the Tuskegee victims? Are there any scenarios that we can create to help us understand what is going on regarding the treatment of Covid-19 patients during this pandemic? Why are some doctors confused, contentious and others confident about the treatment or lack thereof for Covid-19? Which doctors are confused and which doctors are confident about treatment and which doctors feel they

7

The HCQ Debate, Caxton Opere, MD

have to control every narrative about the treatment? What role is the media playing in further fueling this confusion-contention-confidence crisis in the general populace regarding the treatment of Covid-19 and what role have our academic institutions also played? Who controls these academic institutions and why?

These are the questions no one wants to answer without reverting to politics, hocus-pocus, name calling, or other degenerate debate tools. You will have the answers to many of these questions by the time you finish reading *The Hydroxchloroquine Debate: What Did Researchers Hide About Hydroxychloroquine?* By now you can almost be certain that the Hydroxychloroquine debate is probably the single most divisive medical challenge of the modern medical era where there are treatments for virtually everything else.

1

The WHO-NIH Warnings

On January 14, 2020, Dr. Tedros Adhano Ghebreyesus, the Director-General of the World Health Organization, WHO, informed the world in a Tweet that we had nothing to worry about as far as Covid-19 was concerned. Ten days later on January 24, 2020, the top infectious disease physician in the United States and head of the National Institute of Allergy and Infectious Diseases (NIAID), Dr. Anthony Fauci, publicly announced that there was nothing to worry about regarding the outbreak of an unknown viral infection reported in Wuhan China. Turns out that both men were wrong and to this day, it remains unclear why they sent such a message to the rest of the world. These two blunders by the heads of two reputable leading institutions combined may have cost many hundreds of thousands of people their lives and millions their livelihood. . Anyone familiar with contagious diseases knows that when government officials are wearing complete protective gear in January, knows this is something serious enough to warn the world to begin initiating some protective measures. Why would Dr. Tedros (WHO) and Dr. Fauci, (NIAID) not warn the world to prepare and prevent the spread of this highly contagious virus? On an international scale, a decent response would mean warning nearby countries. What's the worse that could have happened if other countries had been warned earlier than March 11? Containment of the virus! The disease that was later called Covid-19 infection would have been drastically curtailed. Yet we are all familiar with hindsight being better than foresight and the consequences of not alerting the nations. Without laying any blame, we still must understand what may be going on behind the scenes. Scenarios can help us understand what may be lurking behind the scenes and how to prepare for what could happen next. So, picture for a moment that you are been transported back in time.

2

$4.5 Trillion Dollar Profit Scenario

You are the CEO of a multi-billion dollar global pharmaceutical conglomerate. You have a few blockbuster drugs in your stalls including an antidepressant, an antipsychotic, a statin for lowering cholesterol, and a painkiller that each bring in billions in sales every year. You also have some other drugs that each bring in several hundreds of millions of dollars every year but the first four above account for almost 85% of your annual revenue. Two of your billion-dollar drug patents are about to expire and you're still battling copycat competitors in court for patent infringements. You're well connected with friends in high government positions, have provided hundreds of millions of dollars in research grants to leading universities, sponsored fellowships, and multiple scholarships for several Heads of Departments in at least ten of the Ivy League universities around the country. Some of those you sponsored are now research professors with worldwide recognition, thanks to your generosity. You've always told your researchers and other employees to read widely beyond their field, look for pain spots in humans and then develop products that would address these pain spots. So far, that has worked out very well for you, your employees and your stockholders. You attended a conference on emerging infections about three years ago that opened your eyes to an entirely new world than the one you thought you knew. On getting back to work, you summoned your Vice President of research and development (R&D), the marketing and publicity team and the head of international clinical research. You shared your new vision with the team and the board members and committed over one hundred million dollars to study emerging pathogens, biological and chemical weapons, develop antidotes, antimicrobials and vaccines. Your goal is to make money from any outbreak.

Ever since computer Mogul Bill Gates' TEDx talk many years ago on a possible pandemic, you had devoted some time to understanding emerging infections. Your scientists had predicted that that the outbreak for a highly contagious and deadly disease with pandemic potential would be in either New York, Washington DC, China or Lagos. You had ears to the ground in these places in case of a deadly outbreak. Things looked promising as you sat down waiting for the next blockbuster drug from your R&D team when Covid-19 suddenly struck. One of your secret scientists in China called you a few minutes after midnight on January 1st, 2020 to tell you that there will be a major outbreak that had already started in China. "This is it" the secret scientist said and ended the call. You had him paid off and made some quick phone calls around the world to your R&D teams. You also called your government contacts, including the CIA head and a few senators. Now you have your scientists working round the clock to identify the virus and begin working to find a cure. You summoned your managers and VP of global affairs, to get a better understanding of what's going on and whatever the competition was doing. No one could give you any new information yet and as you were about to end the meeting, in walks "Prof Einstein". His real name is Donald Raul but he got the nickname for his uncanny ability to nail a problem before the world figured it out. He called out Ebola, West Nile, MERS and a few other outbreaks before the media even let the world know. "What do you think Prof?" you asked the grey-haired head of your virology department and clinical research, also a tenure professor at the local University. He replied by saying "If it's corona we have stuff that could treat it." But why bother spending all our resources when there's a cheap drug out there already. Why re-invent the wheel?" What are you talking about, you responded? Donald was however in the habit of saying things only once, always leaving everyone including the CEO to figure the rest out. He remained silent. Are you saying this is not an opportunity to capitalize upon? "If you want to manufacture a cheap drug that's already sold over the counter in many countries with an expired patent, sure. Our drug treatment will cost thousands and you want to compete against a drug that's cheap and available for only a few dollars? Then you've got work to do," Donald added. While Donald was being sarcastic, you took his words to heart and went to work immediately.

Over the next few weeks, you summoned your marketers, sales people, clinical research leaders, regional vice-presidents and managers to multiple online meetings. You also brought in your propaganda consultant, Boris Cheyenko, a former KGB agent, and a master of brainwashing and advertising techniques. The meeting started with everyone trying to figure out how to compete and capture the Covid-19 treatment market against HCQ, a drug that was cheap and available in almost every country around the world. When Boris arrived and laid down his plan, everyone was shocked. With mouths wide open as he explained that we shouldn't feel sorry for a pill. Here is a portion of what Boris shared with you:

> "By the time we are finished with our campaign against this cheap drug, hydroxychloroquine, no one will want to say the word, no one

11

will want to prescribe it, and even the doctors already prescribing it and getting excellent results, will begin to have doubts. Those who are still strong and have no doubts about using it for treating the coronavirus will either be forced to keep quiet or made to look like fools. We will hire professors and physicians to publish articles denouncing this cheap drug online and in reputable medical journals like the New England Journal of Medicine, Scalpel, London Medical Journal and JAMA, the Journal of The American Medical Association. The only ones who will see through our plan to discredit hydroxychloroquine can be counterattacked using the media and made to look foolish, making them look like they don't know what they're doing. A lot of people may have to die, but those deaths are why people will buy your drugs, Boris concluded, with a sheepish grin. It sounded like a brilliant plan, so you ask Boris, "Will all this work?" and with a smile, Boris' assistant, Ivan, replied, with a thick Russian accent before Boris could respond, "Of course, this is America".

As you began executing Boris' plan over the next few weeks, several medical doctors of repute were contacted and informed that HCQ is ineffective for Covid-19. These doctors believed your company reps even without any scientific data. Many of these doctors had previously received grants, consulting fees and even cruise tickets from your company, so that was easy. Boris had recommended very strongly that as many of these doctors as possible be tainted with gifts so they feel obligated to remain silent. You also called in your accountants and business trajectory experts to help you figure out the potential gains and determine the minimum amount to commit to the entire project. The more you think you're going to make, the more money you can convince the board to allocate to the project. You weren't expecting such a large number from your business and sales experts, but the numbers from four departments in different locations around the world were all in the trillions. According to your most reserved and conservative experts in one department, at $1100 per treatment per person, here is what the expert committee agreed upon to present to the board of directors after meeting with you:

SALES FROM THE COVID-19 MAGIC BULLETS
When they gave you their numbers, you could not believe them. You kicked things up a notch by calling an old friend from high school, Dr. Frank Gambini, who was now head of the World Institute of Health (WIH). After exchanging pleasantries, you shared the cheap vs. expensive drug dilemma with Frank. You promised Frank you'll take care of him if everything goes well. Five days later, while Frank was at a

press briefing with the President of the United States, something changed drastically. It seemed, the President said, that there is a solution to the coronavirus, "something we never thought of before." Frank's heart skipped a beat. While Frank was still hoping this was just a hoax, the President informs Frank that he would like Frank to inform the public about the hope found in this cheap drug HCQ in order to keep the American people encouraged until a cure can be found. The President said he was sure Americans would find a cure, and was in good spirits as he told Frank and the other high-ranking government officials at the Oval Office how he received a phone call from a highly respected virologist from France saying hydroxychloroquine works for Covid-19 and the only thing we have right now. The President would have announced this at the press briefing right after the meeting, but he didn't want to take that honor away from Dr. Frank Gambini. Dr. Gambini on the other hand wasn't too happy about the whole idea of the President figuring out what was effective in treating Covid-19. Telling Frank to announce that to the American people was adding insult to injury. He would not do it. Not with what was at stake and the favor he now owes his friend. Dr. Gambini immediately excused himself to call you. You had just transferred five million dollars into Frank's Cayman account when he called that afternoon to inform you that the President had already found out about the cheap drug from some French virologist and wants to announce the usefulness and safety of the drug. "Well Frank, I trust you to take care of things", you told him. When Dr. Gambini went back in, the meeting was already over and the press secretary had given each speaker a podium assignment. She winked at Frank and told him his job was the easiest as the President said all he had to do was reassure the people we have a safe inexpensive drug that will be made available as quickly as possible. Little did the press secretary know that was the last thing on Dr. Gambini's mind as he managed a stiff half-hearted smile and said, okay. Once on the podium, Dr. Gambini rambled and never mentioned anything about hydroxychloroquine. Furious, the President stepped up to the podium and made the announcement himself. Thus began the hydroxychloroquine debate.

The following weekend you had a game of golf with Jeff, one of your old associates who you had done business with while building your health insurance business. You pair up to play and he said he knows about coronavirus and that while the potential treatment was cheap, it seemed you company was going to make insane profits if you could find a cure. Out of curiosity, you asked your friend how much he was thinking was insane profit. Your friend pulls out his phone and shows you the email

13

he received from his youngest son, a lecturer at Stanford Business School, that morning:

FLAT FEE ESTIMATED PROFITS FROM A COVID-19 MAGIC BULLET:
Estimated cost of treatment per person: $1100
Estimated infected people globally: 100 million
Estimated sales for treating 100 million infected patients
= $1100 x 100 million patients
A = $110 billion

Estimated sales for drug prophylaxis of 1 billion people globally =
$1100 x 1000 million people (1000 million = 1billion)
B= $1.1 Trillion

Estimated sales for vaccine prophylaxis of another 3 billion people =
$1100 x 3000 million people (3000 million = 3 billion)
C =$3.3 Trillion

Total sales $4.51 trillion!

Once your friend showed you this number, you immediately call your head of virology research, told him to culture the virus and start looking for ways to not only treat the virus, but to spread the infection. You would make money from selling your drugs, and you will make sure there is an ever-increasing demand for your drugs, even if it means spreading the infection.

Meanwhile, your good friend Dr. Frank Gambini, is already spreading the idea that the cheap drug is ineffective by refusing to make the announcement as recommended by the President. In surprising despair, the President could not figure out why Dr. Gambini refused to make the announcement and he got up to make the announcement. This was not the plan but the President has no time for slackers. The news went viral. When you saw the news clip on YouTube, you called Dr. Gambini immediately to find out what on earth was going on. He reassured you that his plan A is still effective. To be sure, you arrange a meeting between yourself, Dr. Gambini and Boris, the propaganda and advertising expert. To let Frank know how serious a financial deal this is, you tell him to check his Cayman account. Another five million dollars had been deposited there.

Now that you have this scenario, you should have a better understanding of what follows and what you hear on the news.

Your real name is George Sachs.

3

Enter Dr. Fauci

On Wednesday July 29, 2020, two days after the viral video that featured Dr. Stella Immanuel, Dr. Simone Gold and a few other physicians, Dr. Anthony Fauci, head of the National Institute of Allergy and Infectious Diseases section of the National Institute of Health, came on TV to say "hydroxychloroquine is ineffective". It appeared as if he never wanted those words on his sacred scientific lips, as if the word hydroxychloroquine was an abomination with a bitter taste to the holy lips.

The raging battle began when the US President announced on television that hydroxychloroquine was very helpful in France and appears promising in the treatment of Covid-19. Whether Dr. Anthony Fauci just hated the idea that the President beat him to the announcement in order to be heroic or whether the President took on that role to announce after Dr. Fauci himself had remained mute about this promising drug is yet to be understood or confirmed. If you however analyze the clips and try to put together a scenario in which the head of the National Institute of Allergy and Infectious Disease remained absolutely mute about a promising drug during a deadly pandemic, your mind should start asking questions. If the most influential medical doctor during a pandemic remains absolutely silent about a promising drug, do you think that's a good thing? Particularly when other countries using the drug keep reporting positive outcomes? Was Dr. Fauci hurt by the idea that the use of HCQ was announced by a President with no medical knowledge or was there something else? Politics can get bitter and enviously filled with hatred, but we should never let the lives or livelihoods of millions of people be jeopardized by our egos or political inclinations. Some of us, particularly doctors, have such egotistic depravities that effectively strip us of our humanity. We would rather be right and the patient dead than be wrong while the patient lives. Such sadistic doctors are like the evidence planting district attorneys that boast of never losing a case while condemning innocent people to prison or death row by padding the case. Only this time it is doctors, not district attorneys, sworn to the Hippocratic oath to do no harm, fabricating scientific data to suit their ulterior motives, endangering lives in the process and getting others killed. Above all, some are knowingly rescinding the use of a potentially life-saving drug and gathering pseudoscientific evidence to buttress their deception with statistics, putting entire nations at risk of Covid-19 infection and death.

If there's another reason behind Dr. Fauci's silence on the effectiveness of HCQ in Covid-19, we've not been informed of it yet. You're about to examine some details that should tell you whether those who believe in the drug's effectiveness are doing so out of ignorance or sound medical thinking and practice. You will also be able to decipher if those attacking the drug really do have a sound scientific basis or are driven by a combination of ignorance, political vendetta, a Big Pharma driven profit-based propaganda or an even more sinister plan beyond the reader's imagination. Put on your thinking cap and let's go on a journey that will give you the view on both sides using the very studies that were used to denounce HCQ to reveal the greater truth about this drug. By the time you complete this book, you'll be confident in your decision and well informed about the usefulness, limitations, and uselessness of the studies for and against hydroxychloroquine and arrive at the singular conclusion of whether or not HCQ is effective in Covid-19, regardless of what anyone including Dr. Fauci says. You will then be able to decipher if in fact his July statement was accurate and true or intentionally misleading and false. You will be able to conceive of a number of probable reasons for such deception, if in fact such a deception has occurred. Lastly, whether or not such deception as it affects the lives of the American people by those entrusted with the wellbeing and health of its people, ought to be allowed to go unpunished will be left to you and the justice department to decide.

4

Can Reputable Medical Journals Mislead Doctors?

You bet! In the next few chapters, we will look at some published clinical trials that were used in determining the efficacy or ineffectiveness of HCQ in Covid-19 patients. While many of these clinical trials have been brandished in the news, the substance of what the published articles contain should be clear to healthcare professionals, as it often contradicts what the news says. That's because hiding inside these articles is the fuel for much of the Covid-19-HCQ debate. Every physician needs to thoroughly understand the fundamental problems plaguing these published articles, as they are the driving force behind the hydroxychloroquine debate. Not knowing the flaws in these publications can lead to making the wrong clinical decisions with unintended consequences, the likes of which we are yet to fully appreciate, particularly the medico-legal ones. One thing is sure, if HCQ works for Covid-19 infection, it does change a lot of things economically and socially, provided the right information is allowed in the media.

Many of the research papers on the use of HCQ in Covid-19 are carefully written for the busy physician who needs to quickly browse through a topic or subject and move to the next article or some other task at home or at work. The best peer-reviewed medical journals like the *New England Journal of Medicine* are structured so that a busy physician can open a seven-page article, look through the entire abstract on the first page, read the conclusion in the abstract section and be done with it in seconds. This is the habit retained by busy doctors and practitioners that have chosen the most reliable journal sources such as the *Lancet* or *New England Journal* to update their knowledge and feed their minds. You may be one of these physicians or healthcare professionals. You are about to see how detrimental such a fast and furious approach can be to updating your knowledge or formulating treatment plans and decisions, particularly for Covid-19 patients. On average, a busy practitioner working a 12-hour shift or sometimes more, excluding driving time, has very little time to dissect journal methodology. This practitioner typically picks up a trusted journal and scans the cover for interesting articles. If they find one, they'll likely jump to the abstract section of the article, read its conclusion, and move on. Unfortunately, many of these articles cannot withstand proper scrutiny because they have methodologies and conclusions that have no logical or scientific merit or real world clinical application if carefully read. If only the doctor or healthcare professional browsing these articles would create time to read the sections on "methodology", "results", "discussion" and "comments from other readers" for example, they might discover a goldmine of information that may contradict the conclusion in the abstract section or the title of the paper itself. You will find many such interesting contradictions in this book as you examine several Covid-19 clinical trials. For example, in a May 11, 2020 *Journal of The American Medical Association* article by Rosenberg et al, *(JAMA. 2020;323(24):2493-2502)*, there was no difference in mortality between the treated (HCQ, AZi, HCQ+AZi)and the untreated hospitalized Covid-19 patients. That main body of the text however stated that interpretation of their results may be limited by the very study design itself. In other words, the authors are saying, "don't trust what we say." The take home point from this paper for a busy practicing physician with only a few minutes of browsing would be in one word, confusion. Nothing lends itself to immediate use for the busy practitioner after reading the journal. Even when seeing the same type of hospitalized patients, the journal does nothing useful besides adding confusion to any preexisting knowledge gaps the practitioner had before reading the article. It's as if publishing a COvid-19 paper is a fashion parade or an IQ parade. The mechanics of statistical analysis of a research paper is often beyond the typical practitioner's purvey and so skipping the statistics section reduces the confusion and makes perfect sense. Yet the methodology of the study and results section are too important to ignore as they provide the reader with an understanding and depth that could save them treatment errors of commission or omission, and perhaps preserve their patient's lives and livelihood. My advice would be that if you're not good at analyzing statistics, leave that part alone. Examine the methods and ask yourself if you would have done things the way the authors did it or differently. Then read what other experts critiquing the paper have to say at the end of the paper if such a section exists. The latter comments might shock you and could be a gold mine to help you improve your ability to analyze published papers. I usually don't waste anytime reading the original author's responses to those sometimes scalding letters and comments because it's often a defensive stance, a bunch of excuses, (I'm allergic to excuses), particularly if the critique revealed fatal flaws in the paper. Let's now look at a few of the published journal articles used in deciding the usefulness or uselessness and dangers of HCQ in Covid-19 treatment or prophylaxis.

Coalition Covid-19 Brazilian I Study:
Cavalcanti et al.
Hydroxychloroquine with or without Azithromycin in Mild-to-Moderate Covid-19
New England Journal of Medicine, July 23, 2020
504 patients. Open label, multi-center (55 hospitals)

The first study we will look at is the Brazilian COALITION Covid-19 Study published in the July 23, 2020 issue of the *New England Journal of Medicine* by Cavalcanti et al. The Coalition Covid-19 Brazilian I study is a multi-center, randomized, open-label, controlled study of 667 patients with suspected or confirmed Covid-19 infection. It was designed to assess whether HCQ alone or in combination with azithromycin would be effective in improving clinical status of Covid-19 patients with mild-to-moderate infection at 15 days after hospital admission using a 7-level ordinal scale from 1 to 7 with a higher score implying increased worsening of the patient's condition. 55 hospitals were used to admit patients. The patients were 18 years or older with a mean age of 50 years and 58% were men with suspected or confirmed Covid-19 having symptoms for 14 days or less. They had to be on no more than 4L/minute of supplemental oxygen or less than 40% oxygen by Venturi mask.

The primary outcome 7-level scale used in the study is as follows:
1. Not hospitalized with no limitation on activities
2. Not hospitalized with limitations on activities
3. Hospitalized without supplemental oxygen
4. Hospitalized with supplemental oxygen
5. Hospitalized with supplemental oxygen by high-flow nasal cannula or non-invasive ventilation
6. Hospitalized with mechanical ventilation
7. Death

The study's conclusion in the abstract section of the article states:

> *"Among hospitalized patients with mild to moderate Covid-19, the use of hydroxychloroquine, alone or with azithromycin, did not improve clinical status at 15 days as compared with standard care".*
> *- Cavalcanti et al. 2020.*

The paper provides information meant for three main groups; practicing doctors, national regulatory agencies, and researchers. Regardless of what the article says, the practitioners in outpatient settings claim they are getting excellent results with HCQ alone or in combination with Azithromycin. (HCQ+AZi). Since the pandemic began, National regulatory agencies have been approving HCQ for use in Covid-19 patients in what seemed like a good gesture. Researchers are however publishing observational studies denouncing any benefits of hydroxychloroquine in hospitalized patients. This paper is one of those that made HCQ a villain and casts doubts on the use of HCQ in hospitalized patients. It was the last study that came out days before Dr. Fauci finally blurted out in an MSNBC interview that HCQ is ineffective in Covid-19.

The use of glucocorticoids, other immunomodulators, antibiotic agents, and antiviral agents was allowed in the control group. Hydroxychloroquine was dosed as 400mg twice daily for 7 days and azithromycin as 500mg daily for 7 days. The current standard care for Covid-19 was the physician's discretion and whatever the doctor felt like doing or not doing for their patient. All the trial outcomes were assessed by the site investigators, who were un-blinded, meaning, they were aware of who did or did not receive treatment. A modified intention to treat method was utilized as inclusion of unconfirmed cases would decrease the estimated effect size and power of the study. A total of 42% of the patients were receiving supplemental oxygen at baseline.

> Secondary outcomes included clinical outcome at 7 days (see above); mechanical ventilation within 15 days (number 5); initiation of supplemental oxygen administration (#5 above) from randomization to day 15; duration of hospital stay; in-hospital death; thromboembolic complications; acute kidney injury; number of days alive and free from respiratory support (no supplemental oxygen or assisted ventilation).

Of the 667 patients recruited 504 were confirmed Covid-19. The randomization to the treatment groups followed a 1:1:1 order with the following numbers:

> 229 patients C: Standard care (control group)
> 221patients H: Hydroxychloroquine*
> 217 patients HA: Hydroxychloroquine* + Azithromycin**

* Hydroxychloroquine dose: 400mg twice daily x 7 days
**Azithromycin dose: 500mg daily x 7 days

A total of 18 patients died in the hospital during the study:
    Deaths in the Control group = 6
    Deaths in the HCQ group = 7
    Deaths in the HCQ+ Azi group = 5

Adverse effects in the 3 treatment groups were as follows:
    (C) Control group – 22.6%;
    (H) Hydroxychloroquine – 33.7%;
    (HA) Hydroxychloroquine and Azithromycin – 39.3%

More patients in the HA group had more frequent events of QTc interval prolongation and elevation of liver enzymes.

There are several problems with this study and some of them are underlined in the opening paragraphs above. Remember that the presence of certain specific flaws, sometimes even just one, could completely invalidate a study. Let's look at some of the problems with the study.

Problem #1: "Open-label, controlled."
These two phrases, open-label or controlled should, never be used to describe the same study as they are mutually exclusive. It definitely should not by used professionals publishing a paper in the New England Journal of Medicine (NEJM), one of the world's most prestigious and trusted medical journals. If a study is open-label, then it is not a controlled study. It's unclear why the journal editors accepted this word combination. But lo and behold, there you have it! The Brazilian Coalition Covid-19 study is an open-label controlled study. It's in print, and the addition of the word "control" to the phrase open-label seems to add an air of finality or authenticity to the novice but, who is fooling who? A complete mockery of extremely busy and time-strapped physicians trying to quickly read just the conclusion section of the most trusted medical journal in order to make up-to-date treatment decisions. The Webster's New Collegiate dictionary defines an oxymoron as a combination of contradictory or incongruous words. If you didn't know this, that's okay. If you call your study an open label and yet say it is controlled, well, there's no such thing! It's an insult to busy practitioners and physicians to publish such a paper for the reasons highlighted in the next few paragraphs. If it's blinded it's controlled, if un-blinded, then it's uncontrolled.

21

The HCQ Debate, Caxton Opere, MD

This is what one of the world's foremost authorities on clinical trial designs, Professor Bert Spilker, had to say about open label trials almost thirty years:

> *"Open label trials should not be used in phase I trials conducted in volunteers, phase II pilot trials, phase II pivotal trials, or any other trial in which it is ethically, medically and practically possible to use a double blind design to achieve more reliable data. ...The degree to which a blind is maintained often has a profound effect on data obtained and the interpretation of those data"*
> - Bert Spilker, PhD MD. Guide to Clinical Trials, 1991. Raven Press. New York. p1073.

Open label trials are unacceptable and do not represent strong trials.

Problems #2 & #3: Supplemental Oxygen of 4L/minute in Mild-Moderate Disease

The second problem with the study is that it's not clear what the cutoff point is for starting patients in the study on supplemental oxygen. The third problem is that there is no clear definition of what constitutes mild, moderate or severe Covid-19 infection in this study. I'll take both flaws in the study together. An average clinician who sees patients regularly in the outpatient or hospital setting knows that if they have to place a patient on 4L/minute of oxygen, that patient has become critical or at least severe and probably needs to be in a step-down or intensive care unit, particularly those not responding to initial treatment. Since some patients in this study were not on supplemental oxygen, we can only assume that those who received supplemental oxygen were given oxygen because they needed it, because they were hypoxic. What does that need mean? Let's use four categories of need: those that need 1L/minute, 2L/minute, 3L/minute and 4L/minute of supplemental oxygen by nasal cannula to bring their pulse oxygen saturation to acceptable levels. We don't know what the authors considered to be acceptable levels of oxygen saturation after a patient was placed on supplemental oxygen. Were patients placed on oxygen because of subjective dyspnea, anxiety, respiratory distress or objective hypoxia, tachypnea or acute respiratory failure? One question I would love to ask the study authors is at what oxygen saturation level by pulse oximeter did they start administering oxygen? I'm sure these patients were either hypoxic or in some respiratory distress. Certainly the degree of hypoxia cannot be considered mild or moderate if the oxygen has to be turned up to 4L/minute or the patient is placed on a Venturi mask as was done in the study. While it's not uncommon to start patients with low oxygen saturations by pulse oxymeter on 1-2L/minute of oxygen, such patients usually have an oxygen saturation of 92-94%.

You must also understand that having a low oxygen saturation level due to Covid-19 infection is different from having the same oxygen saturation levels in a patient with only congestive heart failure (CHF), acute asthma or COPD exacerbation. These latter patients have reversible conditions that may rapidly respond to initial treatments, and the patients have probably been in and out of the emergency room several times before. Some of these patients may present with oxygen saturations of 89-90%, but once they receive treatment, sometimes within an hour, may be saturating 98% on room air and insist they're ready to go home. They are sometimes discharged and sometimes observed overnight. If a patient with Covid-19 presents with hypoxia, and is in need of supplemental oxygen, they are probably very severe or critical. On page 47 of *Covid-19: Physician Treatment Strategies*, there is a picture of mild, moderate, severe and critical Covid-19 disease that incorporates both the clinical presentation of oxygen saturation with the ongoing alveolar pathology to help you understand mild, moderate, severe or critical Covid-19 illness. (You can get your copy at the iTunes store or Barnes and Noble, but not Amazon). While not yet tested in prospective randomized placebo controlled double-blinded trials, this picture helps you understand what mild, moderate, severe or critical Covid-19 looks like in the alveoli of the Covid-19 patient and their likely presentation. From this diagram, you'll see that what most people call mild Covid-19 is often severe, and that what they often call moderate is critical or severe. You might have heard anecdotes about young Covid-19 patients with oxygen saturations of 93% suddenly collapsing in front of the doctor or nurse and immediately requiring intubation. Since I work in the emergency room and have treated a few Covid-19 patients, I have found the diagram helpful, as have my nurses and supporting staff. We do not know exactly from this study, what the authors really mean by mild-to-moderate Covid-19 and whether we can go by their classification. We also do not know what their cutoff point is for starting a patient on supplemental oxygen. One thing is clear, if their mild Covid-19 is really severe and their moderate is critical, it may drastically affect their study outcomes and what they're telling us. Low oxygen saturation in a Covid-19 patient is an ominous sign.

One of the classifications of Covid-19 infection described in *Covid-19: Physician Treatment Strategies* uses a perfectly healthy patient with no

The HCQ Debate, Caxton Opere, MD

prior heart or lung disease with an oxygen saturation of 100% on room air now presenting with Covid-19 and on room air, oxygen saturation at any of the following stages:

I =Mild:
O2 Sat 98% or more. Minimal infection. 10% involved lung

II =Moderate
O2 Sat 96-97%. Moderate infection. 20% involved lung

III = Severe
O2 Sat 94-95%. Severe infection. 40% involved lung

IV = Critical
O2 Sat 93% or less. Critical infection. 80% involved lung

Without the oxygen saturation on initial presentation, the use of the mild-moderate classification means absolutely nothing to the clinician trying to find useful application of the study.

Problem #4: No Objective Markers of Severity or Surrogate Markers

Another issue in the COALITION study is the authors failing to discuss their use of surrogate markers or disease severity measurements such as arterial blood gases, arterial pH, lactic acid, cytokine levels or ferritin levels. Several non-research hospital centers now check ferritin levels as a surrogate marker of severity but the authors of the Brazilian COALITION study didn't check such surrogate markers. I think designing a clinical trial of this caliber intending to inform the world about the utility of HCQ without surrogate markers of illness or disease progression for Covid-19 in the 21st century is substandard. So it's still a bit puzzling as to how disease severity was determined particularly in patients receiving oxygen by Venturi mask, even if this was less than 40%. Any experienced critical care physician will tell you that a patient on a Venturi mask is in respiratory failure and critical. Yet the study still classified these patients as mild. In the real clinical situations we encounter, no patient gets to have a Venturi mask that is not severely compromised. It's hard to tell how sick these patients were on admission, particularly those on supplemental oxygen. Many could have been critically ill but wrongly classified as moderate to mild. Gambini?

Problem #5: Late Administration of Hydroxychloroquine

Hydroxychloroquine blocks an early glycosylation step required for the spike protein of the SARS-CoV-2 virus to attach to the ACE-2 receptor of the host cell in the lung. If that process takes place successfully before HCQ is given, the virus attaches to the receptor, enters the cell and can start multiplying. HCQ can still stop this viral replication by increasing the pH of the endosome, the invaginated part of the cell membrane containing the virus particle when it attached to the cell membrane. When the virus attaches to the ACE-2 receptor at the surface of the cell membrane, a reaction takes place and the cell membrane sort of swallows the virus by invaginating into a small ball-like endosome containing the virus. This ball-like endosome carrying the virus needs to decrease its pH in order to release the Coronavirus into the cytoplasm where it can find the ribosome and start replicating. HCQ raises the pH of the endosome thereby preventing release of the virus. As you can see from these steps, HCQ must be given early enough during the course of the infection to be effective. If the endosome releases the coronavirus before HCQ is given, then zinc can inhibit the enzyme responsible for virus replication, RNA- dependent-RNA polymerase.

The study investigators stated that they administered HCQ a median of 7 days from the onset of symptoms and as late as 14 days from onset of symptoms. If hydroxychloroquine were to be effective however, it has to be given early, as many other authors have suggested. For well-informed scientists to give HCQ that late reflects either a flaw in thought process or study design or the Gambini influence. It's a different thing entirely if HCQ is ineffective, but if it is effective, everything points to giving it early. In sepsis and severe pneumonia we expect a patient to get rapid boluses of intravenous fluids and be started on antibiotics early, usually within 60 minutes of arrival or less. In seasonal influenza infection, we expect oseltamivir (Tamiflu®) to be given within 48 hours of onset of symptoms to be most effective. So why did the authors wait 7 to 14 days after the onset of symptoms before administering a potentially effective drug for a deadly disease? It's a violation of first principles. If it could be most effective when given early and patients could die if they fall very ill as a result of unhalted disease progression, why wait that late? The scientific data suggests it should be given early. Rather than admit this was a fatal flaw, the COALITON investigators gave the excuse that their study was better than the Remdesivir study which waited a median 9 days before starting Remdesivir in Covid-19 patients. It's as if this makes the late administration of HCQ acceptable.

The HCQ Debate, Caxton Opere, MD

Problem #6: Dosing of Hydroxychloroquine

The only objective HCQ dosing that we know has received any type of approval (using a panel of experts) is the FDA emergency use authorization (EUA) for HCQ use in Covid-19 given on April 27, 2020 but withdrawn on June 15, 2020. According to the EUA HCQ should be given as
Day 1: 800mg
Days 2-5: 400mg daily
Total = 2.4g

The COALITION Brazil study dosing of HCQ was 400mg twice daily for 7 days and a total HCQ dose of 5.6g. This is more than double the FDA recommended dose of 2.4g over days. It's not clear how this may adversely affect the patient overall, but if the patients were hospitalized for Covid-19, that portends impending respiratory failure or multi-organ failure. Doubling the dose under such circumstances may be more harmful than helpful for patients with impaired oxygenation and cytokine release syndrome.

Problem #7 Adherence

The authors admit that medications perceived as beneficial by both clinicians and patients were not available "despite intense efforts to maintain adherence" and that this resulted in some protocol deviations. How many patients received the complete 7 days of treatment in the treatment groups and how many patients received only a single dose of the treatment drug? Do the authors realize that patients would adhere to the twice-daily in-hospital regimens far better than patients on chronic therapy for other conditions? Do they realize that with patients knowing that Covid-19 infection is potentially life-threatening, they have an automatic incentive for 100% compliance? It is hard to figure out without actual objective parameters how effective the treatment or control groups fared, even among those that received only a single dose of the treatment drug. Efficacy was determined using patients that received only a single dose of the drug. So if a patient received only a single dose of the 14 total doses of HCQ, and was included in the efficacy calculations without any adjustments (what adjustments can you really make if such a patient becomes critically ill), then what exactly are they measuring, a central tendency or a true drug efficacy?

Problem #8 Current Standard of Care at Doctor's Discretion

The current standard of care used in the control group was at the discretion of the physician. That meant the doctor could use anything other than the clinical trial drugs even if what he or she used would introduce significant confounding and therefore confusion. While I'm glad the doctor may have been using treatments helpful to the patients, that open field of treatment is unscientific and does not lend itself to a uniform assessment of the trial outcomes.

Problem #9 Invalidating The Efficacy Study

The biggest misnomer in my opinion, one that probably invalidates the study as a clinically relevant study, is the comparisons made between what the authors call treatment groups versus control group. The study seems as if it was intentionally designed to invalidate the likelihood of any effectiveness of hydroxychloroquine, which is exactly what happened. The study clearly stated that in the control group, patients received glucocorticoids, immunomodulators, antivirals and antibiotics. If you give an immunomodulator to the untreated group, you are nullifying the efficacy you're trying to measure in the drug treatment group, in this case hydroxychloroquine, if that drug treats the illness in question via immunomodulation. It is however an established fact that hydroxychloroquine is an immunomodulator. It is also known by now that the major killing pathway of Covid-19 is hyperstimulation of the immune system which hydroxychloroquine seems to be able to arrest or diminish through immunomodulation and the other two mechanisms, blocking glycosylation and raising endosomal pH.

So if you want to measure the efficacy of HCQ against a control group, you cannot use a control group that is utilizing the very mechanisms that HCQ utilizes in its pathway to mitigate illness. You're invalidating your own study by design. You won't see much difference between the HCQ treated group and the control group. The use of active medicines in the control group is okay to at least ensure the patients do not experience unnecessary hazards of the illness, but doing that invalidates the study trying to measure HCQ's efficacy. Naturally, you wouldn't expect to find a significant difference between the control group on immune modulators and glucocorticoids and those receiving hydroxychloroquine with or without azithromycin in terms of efficacy and this is exactly what the authors obtained. Even more importantly, the fact that active medicines were used in three arms increases the complexity of the results and implies that either

27

1. The medications in all three arms were equally effective
2. None of the medications was effective or
3. It is impossible to determine if any of the three treatments generated any clinical response.

What would have happened if the patients in all three arms had received the same glucocorticoids, immunomodulators and antivirals? Would there have been an obvious difference or an augmentation of HCQ drug effect? Suppose you work in an emergency room and conduct a clinical study on the efficacy of Tdap in tetanus prevention in fresh open wounds. One set will receive Tdap and the other standard care. By standard care you mean thorough wound care, cleaning, antibiotics and pain medications. No one in either group develops tetanus. Can you then conclude that Tdap is not effective in preventing tetanus in patients with fresh open wounds? You can't or rather, shouldn't. Yet, that's what the Brazilian investigators are trying to do with HCQ. Unfortunately they've been able to impress quite a number of people in the USA particularly CNN medical correspondents.

The Brazilian study was unhelpful, weak, inconclusive and perhaps quite misleading, particularly to the majority of physicians who propose and support early administration of hydroxychloroquine in the outpatient setting and avoid hospitalization. One of the accusers of the researchers of this study, Michael James Coudrey, tweeted on April 14,20 2020, claiming they were using the patients as guinea pigs and were irresponsible. Eduardo Bolsonaro, son of the Brazilian President also accused the researchers of being left wing activists in support of the rainbow flag and left wing political candidates and added another political twist to it. Some of these Brazilian researchers received death threats and came under investigation by the federal prosecution team. The question is should they be investigated and who would suggest that they not be investigated for such high doses that ignore the science behind drug toxicity? Lindzi Wessel, writer for the American Association for the Advancement of Science (AAAS) doesn't think such an investigation is justified. But that opinion in her online June 22, 2020 article at AAAS website sciencemag.org titled *"It's A Nightmare." How Brazilian Scientists Become Ensnared in Chloroquine Politics*, Lindzi a writer based in Santiago, Chile, expressed a discontent over the fact that prosecutors were investigating the Brazilian researchers. Such discontent is based on a lack of concern for those that have died, the lost ones they left behind or the reality of scientific thinking. It appears that many journalists writing and attacking pro HCQ doctors, have zero clue why we are in the profession, what the part of a physician is with respect to

28

preventing death and disease, what the phrase off-label means, and what drug toxicity levels mean. The established lethal dose of HCQ, or recommended dosing from other scientists since the onset of the pandemic were completely ignored by the researchers and the investigation is appropriate. If anything, she Lindzi is politicizing an appropriate investigation. It's of note that since the onset of Covid-19 pandemic, many journalists have seen themselves and write as if they are experts on the medical sciences or compassion for the sick and dying. Even if you have a degree in pharmacology or medicine, if you don't have a problem with investigating doctors giving lethal doses of chloroquine to sick helpless patients, then you're part of the problem.

Problem #10: The Study Discussion
The authors admit that the study cannot definitively rule out either a substantial benefit of the trial drugs or a substantial harm. That's because so much was muddled up in the study that it became a sea of chaos. If their assertion is true that they could not rule out any substantial benefit or harm, then why publish it with the intention of providing solutions to the Covid-19 dilemma? It is wrong to outright base decisions that affect the lives of millions on flawed clinical trials with misleading information and false conclusions especially during this pandemic. Nevertheless, Elizabeth Cohen, CNN Medical Correspondent in her online article on July 31, 2020 stated that a "Randomized control trial in Brazil" referring to this same COALITION study we just analyzed, "showed that HCQ doesn't work in hospitalized patients and… a randomized control trial in the United States last month showed it doesn't help prevent infection with Covid-19." It's only appropriate then that the next study we look at is the one journalists seem to love so much, the Bouleware prevention study. Besides these poorly executed and published studies, there is something else brewing in the air. Take a look at the next chapter.

The HCQ Debate, Caxton Opere, MD

6

The HCQ Smear Campaign

Before we look at this next study we'll pull back the curtains briefly to see what's going on with the Big Pharma CEO George Sachs, Boris Cheyenko and Dr. Frank Gambini. All three decided to meet privately to finalize "the plan". Boris explains the plan and every backup that will be needed in case something goes wrong and assures everyone that as long as the right journals are published, doctors won't have time to read them and would agree with whatever is written in the conclusion section without evaluating the methodology or discussion sections. Here is Boris Cheyenko's 17-point Covid-19 Control Plan to make HCQ the most hated drug on the planet:

The 17-Point Cheyenko Covid-19 Control Plan:
- Hook HCQ through the media to a hated celebrity or personality whether dead or alive
- Spread rumors about HCQ's lack of efficacy through media and paid talking heads
- Tell media talking heads to invite doctors for a "honorarium" to say HCQ is ineffective
- Prevent the President from stopping Chinese International flights into the United States
- Avoid interviewing Republicans or anyone that might like the President
- Sponsor sham studies and advertise the studies before the results are published promising carrots on a stick
- Recruit professors with financial and marital problems particularly those paying large alimony sums to conduct clinical trials and pay them extra bonuses up front
- Give toxic and whenever possible lethal doses of HCQ to ensure negative outcomes in the clinical trials
- Announce results of HCQ "failures" in treatment or prevention of Covid-19 using press releases so data and methods can be hidden if necessary
- Avoid peer-reviewed journals and use only press releases for the sham studies where poisonous doses of HCQ are used.
- Get and taint (pay) highly respected professors to endorse the sham studies and denounce the use of HCQ in Covid-19 infections

- Use XNN's 24-hour coverage and other loyal news media outlets to feature and interview several ignorant doctors with key positions and who look good on camera, about HCQ's toxicity and "lack of efficacy"
- Report only Covid-19 infections and deaths and do so every hour of ever day as log as possible until the public say no more
- Avoid reporting recoveries and survivors and block their posts on social media as misinformation
- Do not publish or report any favorable research or success stories on HCQ
- Do not sponsor any debate on pros and cons or efficacy or lack thereof of HCQ
- Do not provide any information through CDC (Center for Disease Control), NIH (National Institute of Health), FDA on how the disease kills for 4 months, so enough people will die from the disease and the rest scared to death of dying

If you've been carefully following the trends, you'd be able to see the execution of this 17-point plan in the news, medical journals, announcements by government officials, press releases and the like.

Let's now look at the clinical trial CNN correspondent Elizabeth Cohen touted as confirming the lack of efficacy of HCQ in Covid-19 and basically nailing the coffin on HCQ.

7

A Randomized Trial of Hydroxychloroquine as Postexposure Prophylaxis for Covid-19
Bouleware, et al. June 2020
New England Journal of Medicine. June 3, 2020
821 patients. Randomized, double-blinded placebo controlled. US + Canada
No face mask or face shield 87.6%
Face mask without face shield 12.4%

821 adults with household or occupation exposure to a Covid-19 confirmed patient were chosen for the study. They had to have been with a confirmed Covid-19 patient at a distance of less than 6 feet for more than 10 minutes while without a facemask or eye shield (high risk) or with a face mask but no eye shield (moderate risk). Patients received placebo or hydroxychloroquine within 4 days of exposure. Patients received 800mg HCQ once followed by 600mg in 6 to 8 hours and then 600mg daily for another 4 days. Exposure was 66% occupational and 34% household-related.

The study reported that the incidence of new illness compatible with Covid-19 did not differ significantly between participants receiving hydroxychloroquine, 49/414 (11.8%) and those receiving placebo, 58/407 (14.3%). The authors concluded that hydroxychloroquine did not prevent illness compatible with Covid-19 infection or confirmed infection when used as PEP within 4 days after exposure.

I find this study quite interesting as it was a randomized, placebo-controlled, double-blinded trial to test the efficacy of HCQ for post-exposure prophylaxis (PEP). At first, it appeared to be a very well designed study from the perspective of gold standard of clinical trials, even though with respect to HCQ and Covid-19, most of these gold standard studies are now looking more like ghost standards.

The study looks great and again any busy practitioner browsing through the abstract section and reading the conclusion will immediately agree with the authors. Until you sit down and carefully examine the details, you may not see the flaws. This time, I'll start with the first five problems, which are responses from other healthcare professionals that read the article and responded to the NEJM editor in the July 15, 2020 letters to the editor.

I'm sure Elizabeth Cohen never read the article itself nor did she read the letters by scientists and medical practitioners such as Dr. Michael Avidan, Dr. Hakim Dehbi, and Dr. Sinead Moretlwe who all agreed that the study had the following problems:

Problem #1: Therapy was given too late
Given HCQ up to 4 days after exposure to SARS-CoV-2 is early treatment not prophylaxis. I couldn't agree more. The study was titled prophylaxis but that wasn't what was carried out. Instead the study was more of preventing symptoms in patients already infected and not prevention of infection.

Problem #2: The study was poorly designed based on #1 above.
The absence of a virologic diagnosis rendered the study useless. Had RT-PCR been done, even if the study was for prevention, it could have given a good idea about early treatment. That opportunity was butchered.

Problem #3: The paper does not prove that HCQ is ineffective in early treatment.

So even though I thought the study was well designed, none of these other doctors felt the design was superb because that's an area where they have some expertise. Again it shows that only trained eyes can come to the right conclusions when looking at a study. So while it might seem as if I'm picking on Elizabeth Cohen, I'm not. I'm just not in favor of people who distort truths that lead to loss of lives as we've experienced during this epidemic and anyone intentionally hiding the truth or distorting it in order to misguide the rest of the world should be held accountable.

Dr. Muhammad Khan and Dr. Javed Butler added one more problem in their letter:

Problem #4: The authors were using the wrong statistical measures to arrive at the wrong clinical conclusions. That is precisely why

> *"Scientific conclusions and business or policy decisions should not be based only on whether a p value passes a specific threshold."*

33

The HCQ Debate, Caxton Opere, MD

-The American Statistician.

The last problem I want to mention from the letters to the editor was from Dr. Babu Tekwani -

Problem#5: Using symptoms to determine Covid-19 infection
You cannot use symptoms alone to prove Covid-19 infection. In some papers for example, just having a headache meant Covid-19! The above 5 problems are sufficient to invalidate any claims or conclusions the study made, but there is more.

Problem #6: Illness Compatible With Covid-19 is not necessarily Covid-19 infection
There are some additional problems associated with the study but because this article was well crafted, the subtleties of what's wrong with the paper could easily escape your conscious mind. For example, the phrase "illness compatible with Covid-19" is not the same as having specific Covid-19 infection. It's easy to miss what the authors did and how they chose to express it.

Problem #7: Calculated Illness of 10% Anticipated Too Low
Investigators anticipating illness compatible with Covid-19 would develop in 10% of patient is not based on established science. SARS-CoV-1 has a basic reproduction number (Ro) of 2.75 and with this virus there was no pandemic. An Ro of 1 or more means that the infected person would infected any person they come in contact with and cause an epidemic in a community if its spread is not curtailed. So with an infection reaching pandemic proportions, the basis for the 10% is unclear and perhaps indefensible based on SARS-CoV-2 having an Ro varying between 2.67 and 5.7. If you come in contact with a SARS-CoV-2 patient and have a high-risk exposure to that person, your risk of getting infected should not be anticipated to about 10% but much higher. First "anticipation" was no longer an issue at the time the study was started in March because as of February 29, 2020, SARS-CoV-2 was already shown to have an Rnought or basic reproductive number of 2.68 (Wu, Leung & Leung, *Lancet February 29, 2020*) and a pandemic had already been declared to a highly contagious and deadly Covid-19 infection. An Rnought of 1 for an infectious agent means that if one person is infected, he or she can spread the disease and cause an epidemic if introduced to a community free of disease. So when you get Ro numbers as high 5.7 from the CDC's publication *Emerging Infectious Diseases (Volume 26, Number 7)* you cannot anticipate a 10% infection rate with close contacts.

The infection rate will be close to 100% if not higher, based on SARS-CoV-2's Rnought. But there's more.

Problem #8: Patients were not tested for Covid-19 Infection before starting HCQ Prophylaxis

Think that's impossible? You would think! Yet, that's exactly what these authors did. The authors admit they did not test many of the subjects before starting them on HCQ as prophylaxis. If you really want to know the truth about HCQ's efficacy in preventing Covid-19 infection, wouldn't you test the high-risk subjects for infection first, to see if they already have the infection, before starting them on prophylaxis? It's obviously no longer prophylaxis if you give them a drug after they're infected. Otherwise how do you prove that HCQ is not effective in Covid-19 prophylaxis if you gave it to patients that were already infected with the virus? You are doing the wrong study! Yet the study investigators stubbornly kept at it, knowing they were doing the world a great injustice by publishing data saying HCQ does not prevent infection. Healthcare workers fully protected but within a few seconds of a small error in exposure can get infected. How much more subjects who were at close contact, less than 6 feet away and for more than 10 minutes with a confirmed Covid-19 case, as were recruited into the study. You can be sure that 99% of such individuals were already infected with Covid-19 based on the Ro of SARS-CoV-2 of 5.67. Many were never tested. Intentionally? You decide. You would think that the authors should have taken into consideration the importance of this particular study, which I think could have been one of the most important clinical trials of the year if not the century. Here are at least five reasons why this could have been the most important clinical trial of the year, had it been properly conducted:

1. Fear elimination. Everyone is afraid of Covid-19, but if this study were done right and proves HCQ was effective in prophylaxis, no one would be afraid anymore.
2. Freedom. People would be free to move around and do business without the lock down
3. Financial setbacks would have been self-imposed not lockdown imposed.
4. Faith in the healthcare system and government would have remained high
5. Our lives and livelihoods restored back to normal

The HCQ Debate, Caxton Opere, MD

None of these things happened, and instead we have the exact opposite, pervading fear, fractured freedoms, financial setbacks and destruction of economies of many nations, and Americans losing faith in the healthcare system and government officials. Not to talk of doctors afraid of prescribing the only helpful drug in outpatients with Covid-19 infection.

Problem #9: Toxic Loading Dose

According to a WHO publication, a dose of 1.5g of chloroquine could be lethal. Doses approaching 1.5g would therefore be accompanied by side effects, mainly gastrointestinal or even cardiovascular and neurological ones such as nausea, vomiting, weakness and dizziness. Study participants in the Bouleware study received an initial dose of 800mg HCQ and another 600mg six to eight hours later. While not lethal, this total of 1.4g in 6 hours was more than 50% of the total 2.4g FDA recommended HCQ dosing over a 5-day period. The FDA recommended dosing allowed 1.2g in 24 hours while this Bouleware 1.4g HCQ was given over 6 hours! Toxicity factor here would be multiplied by four in those six hours!

Problem #10: Inconsistent Dosing Regimen for Patients with Adverse effects

Authors basically informed patients to divide the pills into two or three doses as they saw fit if they had side effects. Almost a quarter 22.9%(80/349) had nausea or upset stomach, 23.2%(81/349) had diarrhea, abdominal discomfort or vomiting. These patients were not under any direct observation to ensure they took the pills. The only real incentive asides from cash incentives was probably the fear of death from Covid-19, which was a good one anyway. There was however no consistent approach to handling subsequent dosing that would be uniform in all subjects experiencing side effects from treatment. A keen observer might easily conclude that the study was designed to have a negative outcome with respect to HCQ's efficacy.

Problem #11: Study Sponsor Conflict of Interest

The study was sponsored by Dr. Fauci's National Institute of Allergy and Infectious Disease and if you read my second book on Covid-19, COVID-19: Physician Treatment Strategies, you'll see how government institutions in the United States, with the exception of the President of the United States, had failed us all. Dr. Anthony is anti-HCQ for whatever reasons. He is known to say very often he uses "science and data" but if this study is one of the "science and data" papers he uses, there's a huge problem. This study is also a CNN favorite, cited by its correspondents.

Problem #12: Downplayed Efficacy of HCQ

All the above problems were enough to sabotage any efficacy attributable to HCQ but the authors made sure they downplayed any positive effects of HCQ. As you would see in the chapter on UNFAVORABLE STATISTICS, the efficacy of HCQ is often downplayed while its companion, or rather, competition, Remdesivir, is often glorified with similar numbers. In the Bouleware study, the incidence of new illness in the HCQ group was 11.83% (49/414) and 14.25% (58/407) in the placebo group. The investigation authors downplayed the 2.42% difference in favor of HCQ.

Problem #13: Only 15% tested positive for SARS-CoV-2

Of the 107 patients that were presumed to have developed Covid-19 infection in the study, only 16 of them were tested and positive for SARS-CoV-2. What kind of standard accepts 15% of anything as a passing grade? Not the NIH I used to know. Nevertheless, this study played an extremely important role in deciding on the recommendations for pre-exposure prophylaxis (PrEP) and post-exposure prophylaxis (PEP) by the expert panel on Covid-19 Treatment guidelines August 27, 2020 update. How did that happen?

The initial loading dose in the Bouleware et al study was too high. If adverse effects to medication were intentionally used in the design to deter treatment adherence according to the Gambini plan, the next study goes to the extreme. While the total dose in Bouleware's study was only 58% higher than the FDA recommended HCQ dosing, the next study by Bourba et al is an interesting one.

8

CLOROCOVID-19
Borba et al
Effects of High vs. Low Doses of Chloroquine Diphosphate (CQ) as Adjunctive Therapy for Patients Hospitalized With Severe Acute Respiratory Syndrome Coronavirus 2 (SAS-CoV-2) Infection
JAMA Network, Open Access. April 24, 2020
81 patients, parallel, double-masked, randomized, Single center, 18 years or older

Hospitalized patients were 18 years or older with a respiratory rate greater than 24/minute, heart rate greater than 125/minute in the absence of fever, and/or peripheral oxygen saturation lower than 90% on room air, and/or an arterial pressure lower than 65mm Hg (shock) with the need for vasopressors, oliguria or lower level of consciousness. Subjects were enrolled regardless of confirmed etiology. Chloroquine phosphate, (CQ) the more toxic form was used in this study. One group of patients, the high dose group, received 600mg twice daily for 10 days. The second group received the modified FDA version of chloroquine phosphate 450mg twice daily on day 1 and 450mg daily on days 2-5. Not too surprisingly, the study was terminated on day 13 of enrolment because of dangerous toxicities. By day 13 of enrolment, 6 of 40 (15%) patients in the low dose group had died compared with 16 of 41 patients (39%) in the high dose group. The data safety monitoring board (DSMB) therefore terminated the study after only 81 patients had been enrolled for the clinical trial. There was prolongation of QTc in 4 of 36 (11.1%) patients in the low dose group and 7 of 37 (18.9%) in the high dose group. Three of 5 patients (60%) in the high dose group with underlying heart disease died.

Based on the pathophysiology of Covid-19, we know it is important to start early treatment for SARS-CoV-2, directing treatments at cytokine production. Waiting till patients require hospitalization means you have waited too late.

Problem #1: Toxic doses of CQ were administered to patients and justified the higher dose while ignoring the available science on in-vitro studies as well as the combined multiplier effect of reduced excretion of CQ in patients with shock as well as the pro-arrhythmic effect of high levels of cytokines in severe Covid-19 infections.

Problem #2: Dosage recommendations from the Brazilian Ministry of Health Ignored

The Brazilian Ministry of Health recommended lower doses, but the study investigators used toxic doses, with the patients as guinea pigs.

Problem #3. No EKG's were performed on patients with elevated CPK 39.4% (13/33) or elevated CKMB 38.4% (10/26). So it didn't seem as if the goal was to take care of these sick patients. Even a medical student knows that an elevation of these two enzymes means you should at least get an EKG to rule out myocardial infarction. Did they measure troponin levels? That would depend on the goal! Nevertheless the study which was reported in the *JAMA Network Open April 24,* 2020 journal showed that the high dose of chloroquine phosphate 600mg given twice daily for 10 days may have been toxic with greater CK elevations in this group than those receiving 450mg daily from day 2 to day 5 days after an initial 450mg twice daily on day 1. CQ causes a myopathy and in patients hospitalized and placed on ventilators who develop myopathy from an overdose of CQ, the likelihood of recovery from that myopathy or coming off the ventilator is very slim. A true Boris Cheyenko effect?

Problem #4: it's very likely that the ventilator plug must have been pulled on many patients that would have survived, had they not received toxic doses of myopathy-inducing chloroquine.

The high dose group received a total of
600mg twice daily x 10 days
= 12000mg
= 12g

The low dose group received
450mg x 2 doses on day 1 + 450mg daily from days 2-5
= 900mg +1800mg
= 2700mg
= 2.7g
This latter with a total CQ of 2.7g was the dose recommended by the Brazilian Ministry of Health based on expert opinion.

It's still puzzling why the authors of this study would use such high doses of chloroquine phosphate (CQ), particularly after the study published by Yao, Zhang & Cui et al in the **March 9, 2020** issue of the journal **Clinical Infectious Disease.** Yao et al recommended doses that were very close to what was used safely in clinical scenarios with HCQ:

Recommended HCQ dosing (Yao et al, 2020)
400mg bid on day 1
200mg bid day 2 – 5 (400mg x 4)
= 2g total dose of HCQ

Recommended CQ Dosing (Yao et al, 2020)
500mg bid x 5 days
= 5g total dose of CQ

Problem #5: Three QTc prolonging agents given simultaneously to critically ill patients

The critically patient with Covid-19infection has high levels of cytokines. High cytokine levels are pro-arrhythmic and such patients are at risk of developing potentially lethal arrhythmias. To then add three pro-arrhythmic agents into the bloodstream almost guarantees a disaster. QTc prolongation, an abnormality that can trigger a deadly malfunction of the heart's normal rhythmic pace, is often drug induced but may be congenital or acquired. It may precede arrhythmia development in patients taking chloroquine phosphate, azithromycin or oseltamivir as all three drugs individually can prolong the QTc interval. When two or more of these three drugs are combined, the effect on QTc prolongation may be minimal, multiplied or malignant. In this Borba et al study, 100% of the patients received azithromycin, 86.8% (33/38) of the patients in the low-dose CQ treatment group received oseltamivir, and 92.5% (37/40) of the high high-dose CQ group received oseltamivir. The combination of all three, that is chloroquine phosphate, azithromycin and oseltamivir, could be deadly, particularly toxic to the hearts of patients with severe covid-19 infection. Not too surprisingly, 39% (16/41) patients receiving high dose CQ (12g) died compared with 15% (6/40) in the lower dose (2.7g) by day 13.

Giving high dose chloroquine phosphate to severely ill Covid-19 patients can increase the risk of death. To give triple therapy (three QTc prolonging agents) certainly guarantees a poor outcome in sick patients.

These were the additional treatments patients in the Borba et al study received:
IV Ceftriaxone 1g twice daily x 7 days (all)
IV Azithromycin 500mg daily x 5 days (all)
Oseltamivir 75mg twice daily x 5 days (most)

Problem #6: No Placebo Control group

Problem #7: Small sample size
It's hard to extrapolate findings from a small study without sufficient power to a larger population.

Problem #8: Letter by Judith Jacobi to the authors
In her letter to the authors, Judith Jacobi, a pharmacist, mentioned the 500mg CQ phosphate twice daily for 10 days used in China, equivalent to a total of 6g CQ base. Borba et al used double this CQ base, a total of 12 g. Toxicities cannot be avoided under those circumstances.

Problem #9: Chloroquine phosphate dosing vs. Chloroquine base dosing not understood.
It possible that Borba et al confused chloroquine phosphate dosing with chloroquine base dosing.

Let's visit Dr. Gambini, to see how much progress he is making with the Boris Cheyenko plan.

Dr. Frank Gambini, head of the WIH, calls some of the grant recipients from the WIH to chit chat with them briefly while subtly hinting them that hydroxychloroquine is ineffective in Covid-19 and that he would like to see more studies showing it's lack of efficacy. He also hinted these researchers some of them University professors, that the WIH will be funding such studies with a fast track for grant approval. He also advised them that if they could not get their clinical trials published in reputable journals, the media will rally behind them and do a press release. Frank reminded them that the goal is to make a lot of noise about HCQ's lack of efficacy in the hospitalized patients. He knew media brainwashing techniques perfected by Boris will make most doctors start thinking and believing HCQ really lacks any efficacy even in outpatients. Since then, two highly publicized studies were stopped early as the authors claimed there was no benefit to hydroxychloroquine. One was the ORCHID study(HCQ x 5 days vs. placebo) and the other was SOLIDARITY (HCQ vs. standard care). Both were stopped early due to little or no benefit of HCQ in hospitalized patients. The results of these studies were shared in "press releases".

The HCQ Debate, Caxton Opere, MD

9

Covid-19 and My Carpenter's Thumb

Forty-five year old John Carpenter was just admitted to the intensive care unit when you came on your shift. Everything started with a small splinter of wood at work. He had removed the splinter that **pricked** his thumb and had continued working. The next day he was feeling a little pain and called his doctor. He was given an appointment to come in the very next day and he did. The doctor did his annual physical and told him to pay close attention to any changes and that the hand didn't look infected. The next morning he noticed some **pain** but he had a busy day at work. By nighttime he noticed the pain was accompanied by **redness** and increased swelling of the thumb. He called his doctor's office and they told him to simply dip the thumb in salt water and come in if that wasn't helping. By the next morning, the swelling and pain had increased substantially and it looked like there was a large well rounded mass on the thumb. John saw his doctor that morning and was told he had an **abscess**. The doctor prescribed an antibiotic ointment for him to rub over the abscess. The next day, John had **chills and a fever** and went back to his doctor. John was given an antibiotic prescription, told to start using it right away and while he was waiting in line at the pharmacy, collapsed on the floor. When he arrived in the emergency room via ambulance, he was told he was in **septic shock** with a blood pressure of 80/42, a temperature of 101.4°F, a heart rate of 126/minute, all from the large abscess on his right thumb with a swelling extending to his wrist. When the primary care doctor was later informed of John's admission to the ICU, he said the "antibiotic ointment was ineffective". Does that sound familiar? Let's break down what happened here that almost cost John his life and what could have been done differently. How does this apply to Covid-19? By staging what happened to Mr. Carpenter, you'll grasp what is going on with him and what the doctor who first saw him in the clinic could have done differently to prevent this outcome. Doing this will help you understand the best approach to managing Covid-19.

Stage 1: Pricked by wooden splinter. Bacteria introduced

Stage 2: Pain from early mild infection

Stage 3: Redness from cellulitis

Stage 4: Swelling of thumb and hand from abscess

Stage 5: Sepsis with chills and fever

Stage 6: Septic shock and death if not properly treated

At stage 1, properly cleaning the wound after John removed the splinter of wood may have sufficed. He didn't. This led to Stage 2, where early signs of infection where then accompanied by later signs of cellulitis and then an abscess. When he had pain and redness (Stage 3, the doctor could have started him on oral antibiotics and given him a tetanus shot, but didn't. When the abscess was diagnosed (Stage 4), the doctor could have incised the abscess and started John on oral antibiotics. That didn't happen either. The doctor told him to rub an antibiotic ointment on an abscess. Not funny! By the time John started having chills and fever (Stage 5) he was experiencing the signs and symptoms of a spreading systemic infection. When he collapsed from septic shock, he could have died (Stage 6). Imagine the ER doctor's response when she told John's primary care doctor that John was admitted for septic shock and he responded by saying "the antibiotic ointment was ineffective". Does it make any sense to give an antibiotic ointment to a patient in stage 4 or septic shock from an abscess and then tell the world that antibiotic ointments don't work? Shouldn't the world also be asking - "when does it not work?" You cannot give a man who needs antibiotics and abscess drainage an ointment and expect it to work. You don't wait until it is too late to give a patient a drug at stage 4 what you should have given it to them at stage 1 or 2 and then blast it all over the news that the same drug is ineffective. Yet every single day, that's what many researchers are doing through their publications on HCQ's lack of efficacy. HCQ has been shown to be effective clinically in hundreds of thousands of patients with Covid-19, pharmacologically both in-vitro and in vivo, and in several contradictory clinical trials, contradictory because the published clinical trials stating HCQ is ineffective actually prove that they don't know if it works and admit it may still be. What's more, HCQ has also been shown to have not just clinical and pharmacological efficacy, but stereotactic efficacy *(Fantini et al, 2020)* at the molecular level. You will see more about the molecular dynamics between SARS-CoV-2, HCQ and azithromycin, in the latter part of chapter 17. Covid-19 is staged a little differently here just to drive home a point of how the puncture wound analogy fits Covid-19 infection closely. Covid-19 Stage 1 is **Exposure (Puncture)**; Covid-19 Stage **2** is **Early (Pain)**; Stage **3** is **Mild** infection **(Cellulitis)**, Stage 4 is **Moderate (Abscess)**; Stage **5 Severe (Sepsis, Fever)**; Stage 6 is Critical (Septic shock). Just like an antibiotic ointment would work on John Carpenter at stages 1-3 but not 4-6, HCQ works effectively at stages 1, 2 and 3 but not at 4, 5 or 6. So why are studies been done using HCQ in stages 4,5 or 6? And why are all the studies done using HCQ at stages 1,2 and 3 (Bouleware et al, Skipper et al) presenting misleading conclusions in their abstracts while admitting the studies were flawed in the body of their text? Why is the government using these flawed trials to formulate recommendations and calling them AIII level recommendations? Gambini's influence?

If you go to the www.cdc.gov website and click on Coronavirus Disease (Covid-2019). Scroll down to "Health Care and Public Health" and click on "Healthcare Professionals" then click on "Clinical Care", Therapeutic Options and "interim guidelines for the medical management of COVID-19 and click "VIEW GUIDELINES". Scroll down to the August 27 Update showing Key Updates to the Guidelines. You'll see where the *Covid-19 Treatment Guidelines Panel* (C19TGP) recommends against the use of HCQ and CQ for the treatment of Covid-19 in hospitalized (Stages 4-6 only for this chapter, and I totally agree) and non-hospitalized patients (Stages 1-3, and I totally disagree) except in clinical trials. These recommendations are dubbed AIII. Then scroll down a little further and click on "Prevention and Prophylaxis of SARS-CoV-2 Infection". You'll then see that the (C19TGP) recommends AGAINST THE USE OF ANY agents for SARS-CoV-2 for pre-exposure or post-exposure prophylaxis and dubbed the recommendations AIII. Both the AI and AIII recommendations were based on the Bouleware et al and Mitja et al studies in chapters 7 and 21 respectively. You will be puzzled as to why on earth these studies were even considered in making such broad-brush reckless uncaring recommendations that override commonsense and the skill, judgment and training of intelligent physicians. The Gambini factor of course!

Rating of Recommendations: A = Strong; B= Moderate; C= Optional
The only strong recommendation from the NIH is the one preventing the use of HCQ/CQ in hospitalized patients. Even then, patients, depending on their stage (3 or 4) may be hospitalized at the last leg of efficacy of HCQ and still show some response particularly when adjuncts such as zinc are included. Who will sponsor such a study?

Rating of Evidence
I = One or more randomized trials with clinical outcomes and/or validated laboratory endpoints.
II = One or more well-designed nonrandomized trials or observational cohort studies
III = Expert Opinion

10

ORCHID

**(Outcomes Related to Covid-19 treated with HCQ
Among In-patients with Symptomatic Disease)
Multicenter, blinded, placebo controlled
479 adults 18 or older, 34 US hospitals. Total HCQ 2.4g**

479 adult patients hospitalized with Covid-19 in 34 US hospitals over an 11-week period. Multicenter blinded, placebo controlled, randomized trial sponsored by the NIH. Patients received either HCQ for 5 days or Placebo. HCQ dosing was 400mg bid on day 1 and 200mg bid on days 2 to 5. The study was conducted by the *Prevention and Early Treatment of Acute Lung Injury (PETAL)* arm of the NIH.

We can expect that with the influence Dr. Frank Gambini has, a study sponsored by the NIH will be influenced and exploited to the maximal possible effect. That means the study will be stopped suddenly, the results will be shared in a press release not a peer-reviewed journal. In peer-reviewed journals, many brilliant minds will lodge complaints about the flaws in any study, sometimes to devastating effect. So since the retracted Mehra study backfired, Gambini's people would prefer press releases. Of course, when a clinical trial is stopped, the public feels the doctors were doing the most compassionate and right thing and it makes the investigators look really good to the public. Details of the exact methodology, flaws, and statistical analysis of the ORCHID will probably remain a mystery and could not be identified as the authors used press releases (Gambini style) not peer-reviewed journals. Using press releases guarantees that no intelligent criticism of the article or clinical trial is going to ever occur. This is a study conducted by Dr. Fauci's NIH.

Study was stopped due to lack of benefit and announcements reported in VUMC News and Trial Site News. According to a VUMC Reporter, Dr. Wesley Self, an emergency physician at Vanderbilt University Medical Center and lead investigator was quoted as saying "Hydroxychloroquine is not a useful treatment for adults admitted to the hospital with Covid-19." Dr. Self is partially right that HCQ is not useful

45

in hospitalized Covid-19 patients and shouldn't be expected to, at least from what we've known for some time now. HCQ is supposed to prevent toxic cytokine buildup and really should be given at the earliest stages of Covid-19 infection in outpatients. That's because by the time a patient requires hospitalization, it is often too late to give HCQ, even though a few patients may still benefit from it. I shared more about when best to use HCQ in Covid-19 infection in my book *Covid-19: Physician Treatment Strategies*. If you read the book, it's been out since May 2020, you won't expect any real benefit from HCQ administered to hospitalized severely ill Covid-19 patients in the fourth or fifth phase of this deadly illness. Even then, Dr. Self's generalization can't be true for all hospitalized Covid-19 patients. As you'll see later on in other studies mentioned in this book, it'll be illogical to hypothesize that all hospitalized patients will not benefit from HCQ. How did Dr. Self arrive at such a non-scientific conclusion? As the scenario showed, if the goal was to make HCQ look really bad that no doctor would ever want to pronounce the drug's name, much less prescribe it, then, the con is on already.

Problem #1: The study is under the control of a biased leader, Dr. Anthony Fauci.
Dr. Anthony Fauci cannot deny his dislike for HCQ. He always seemed very hesitant to mention that hydroxychloroquine may have a use in Covid-19 infection. I'm not sure he ever mentioned the drug until July 29, 2020 when he finally blurted out that hydroxychloroquine was ineffective. I equally suspect that he and a few others know how truly effective HCQ is in Covid-19 infections. Nor do I think he would mention publicly that Covid-19 is a cytokine disorder that even without a cure, can be treated with excellent or reasonable outcomes by blocking cytokines or other molecular mechanisms responsible for the deaths in Covid-19 before they exceed a cutoff point, despite all the science and data available to enable him do so.

Problem#2: ORCHID was stopped and results "press released".
No peer-reviewed publication, and that is beginning to look more like a classic Gambini move. The NIH released a media advisory on Saturday June 20, 2020 stating NIH HALTS CLINICAL TRIAL OF HCQ. Study shows treatment does no harm, but provides no benefit the subheading declared. The NIH has release only few press releases on a Saturday! With what you now know about published studies from the last few chapters, you can't reasonably accept any news over the phone or from a press release as authentic. Yet I listen to doctors who show from what they say that they only listen to the news about HCQ or read only the

conclusion section in the abstract part of the entire journal article they may be referencing.

Problem #3: Wrong Patient Group Studied for HCQ's Efficacy
Patients studied were hospitalized and probably late in the course of the disease, too late for HCQ to have any effect. It makes no sense to start such a study in hospitalized patients when the goal ought to be to find an effective early treatment rather than waste resources and lives trying to prove that HCQ doesn't work for Covid-19 patients. It's clear that this study should equally have attempted a prophylactic arm as well as an early treatment arm. If you however recall the scenario in chapter one, you know that's never going to happen. There's never going to be a useful study that intelligently looks at the efficacy of HCQ in Covid-19 in the United States, as long as Dr. Frank Gambini can have his way.

Here are at least two comments about ORCHID that I found on a website www.trialsitenews.com .

Ken Kremesec on June 28, 2020 said

"Disgusting. HCQ with zinc has been proven effective when used in the early stages over and over. Why do the media and search engines manipulate or hide the data indicating the positive results? Is it because there is so much money to be made via a vaccine?"

Mark on June 23, 2020
"So they used an antiviral at a late stage when what was needed was anti-clotting and immune dampening to prevent the cytokine storm. If NIH can't figure out treatments any better than this, we are in trouble. Use HCQ early when the viremia is peaking. Seems simple enough, why can't they understand this. So disappointing and dangerous that they have failed at such a simple concept."

The HCQ Debate, Caxton Opere, MD

RECOVERY
Randomized Evaluation of CoVid-19 thERapY
Horby, et l
11,303 patients. United Kingdom
Sponsors: Bill & Melinda Gates Foundation, Wellcome, UK Government

11,303 patients from 176 NHS hospitals in the UK randomized to different treatments on a platform study with a single end point, death within 28 days. Patients received one of the following four treatments or to usual care: dexamethasone, hydroxychloroquine, lopinavir-ritonavir or azithromycin. Patients would then be randomized to either receive no further treatment or convalescent plasma. Those with worsening Covid-19 infection could be randomly assigned to receive no further treatment or to receive tocilizumab. Dexamethasone was a success and hydroxychloroquine a failure. But this should not come as a surprise. The age-adjusted mortality rate ratio for dexamethasone compared with usual care was 0.83 (95% CI 0.75-0.95; p<0.001) with an absolute mortality benefit of 2.8%. Today, many physicians would recommend and give dexamethasone based on this study. This is an important breakthrough. The adjusted mortality benefit in patients on mechanical ventilation for dexamethasone was 0.64 (95% CI, 0.51-0.81) with an absolute mortality benefit of 12.1% (remember that HCQ is not for patients on ventilators but to prevent patients from getting on ventilators!)

Problem #1: Toxic dosing of HCQ Reached Lethal Dosing Limits
This is how HCQ was dosed for those poor patients in the HCQ arm:
HCQ 800mg at time zero;
HCQ 800mg 6 hours after first dose;
HCQ 400mg 12 hours after the first dose
HCQ 400mg 18 hours after the first dose

This comes to a total of 2.4g in 18 hours! The patients received 1.86g within 24 hours, 24% more than the lethal dose of 1.5g. The poor patients succumbed. As deadly as the virus was in untreated patients, those who received HCQ had a higher mortality. In the HCQ arm of the study, 1,561 patients received HCQ while 3,151 received usual care. The 28-day mortality for HCQ was 25.7% and for usual care 23.5% with no statistical difference (p=0.1) even though Statnews.com did highlight this slight difference and called it an 11% higher mortality difference against HCQ. The results of the study were shared on Tweeter by the lead authors according to www.statnews.com's Matthew Harper on June 5, 2020. Sound familiar? One of the main reasons for this discrepancy was the toxic or lethal dosing of HCQ. Sounds like the Cheyenko plan at work!

Problem #2: HCQ Dosing Used in the Protocol Deleted without a Trace from the Website

Shortly after the study showed a higher mortality in the HCQ group, the chief investigator Tweeted the results as well as the link to the protocol for the study. (Tweeter, Gambini, press release, sounds familiar?). Trouble started when one observer on Tweeter noticed that the doses given to the HCQ group were highly toxic and perhaps lethal and pointed it out to the Professor on Tweeter. Some drama ensued and the protocol disappeared. The protocol reappeared subsequently on the RECOVERY trial website, only this time there was no sign that HCQ was ever used in the study. You have to go back several dates to find the original dose. Patients died in this study due to lethal doses of HCQ and evidence that HCQ was ever used in the study was carefully hidden away.

Problem #3: Acclaimed Professors Seemed to Love the Outcome in The HCQ Arm

It's bad enough that the RECOVERY study was looking like the Tuskegee study in its HCQ arm, but to have professors from leading institutions in England like Cambridge University or Imperial College, confidently ignore this level of atrocity and begin to vilify HCQ is absolute shameful. The comments from these professors demonstrates a complete disregard for human life, assuming that they know the lethal dose of chloroquine. Endorsing the study or even associating with it is baffling. It's the equivalent of approving a study in which helpless little kids from poor families are allowed to eat peeling lead paint and studied for the neurological effects of lead poisoning over time. I suspect there's a Gambini factor involved here because this is a very odd behavior for British professors.

As there was no peer reviewed publication or data on the HCQ arm of the study, finding information on it was hard. I eventually recovered

49

some information from the science media center online. There, several notable English professors and one doctor working for the pharmaceutical giant Wellcome, voiced their opinion regarding hydroxychloroquine's role in the RECOVERY study in the June 5, 2020 www.sciencemediacenter.org webpage. Some of these professors however jumped to conclusions with extrapolated ideas and biases and failed to conduct thorough analysis of the HCQ study arm. For example, **Professor Stephen Evans,** Professor of Pharamcoepidemiology at the *London School of Hygiene and Tropical Medicine (LSHTM)* was reported on the website as saying:

> *"It will be good to have confirmation from the other randomized trials involving hydroxychloroquine to show that it does not have benefit in treatment, and to be able to characterize that it is equally of no benefit given early or late in the course of illness."*

When a professor of pharmacoepidemiology at the *London School of Hygiene and Tropical Medicine* is praying and hoping that a cheap, inexpensive, readily available drug with an excellent safety profile for over six decades will fail, you can almost bet that's the Gambini plan at work. If it's hard for you to appreciate the depth of knowledge, experience and reputation of a Professor of pharmacoepidemiology at the world-renowned LSHTM if you've never been in that world, I'll help you a little bit. In the United States, anyone can be called a professor if they lectured in the university. In England, you must earn the title "Professor". You will teach, present at meetings and conferences, publish research papers usually for more than a decade after getting your PhD, before you can earn the title of reader and then eventually get promoted to professor. By that time, you're probably going to be recognized by the entire University system as a brilliant hardworking individual with an uncanny attention to detail. As a professor, there is nothing that you will overlook in your field, and your students and colleagues alike will have the utmost respect for you because of the almost encyclopedic knowledge at your fingertips in your field of expertise. I was taught by these types of professors in medical school, many of them British trained, and they cannot overlook the toxic doses of HCQ given to patients in the RECOVERY study. What's even more amazing is that the LSHTM professors are a unique breed of thorough professors whose knowledge and repute is astonishing. They train doctors, nurses, pharmacists, and clinical trial experts from around the world, as well as local healthcare workers and dispensary workers in many villages in developing countries. LSHTM professors are not just verse in their field, they are world class, and have a lot of contact with different cultures from around the world regularly. In other words, while a professor in the UK is highly esteemed, a professor at the LSHTM is a very special breed of intellectual power and influence. An LSHTM professor is definitely not the type that would miss the toxic or lethal hydroxychloroquine doses given to patients in the RECOVERY study. The professional certification course in pharmacoepdiemiology and pharmacovigilance at the London School of Hygiene & Tropical Medicine is a 30 credit, 300-hour didactic course with 80 hours formal teaching, 120 hours of self-directed study, and 100 hours of project time. One would also have to assume that Professor Evans never read the study by New York University's Dr. Carlucci or Henry Ford Hospital System's paper by Dr. Zervos. He just went for the bait. **Professor Peter Openshaw**, (*Experimental Medicine*) agreed that HCQ is of no value in hospitalized Covid-19 patients but added a little Gambini to it when he was quoted on the website as saying

> "*this clearly tells us that HCQ is not to be used in "those" with COVID-19".*

By "*those with Covid-19*", one may safely presume Professor Openshaw meant hospitalized Covid-19 patients. Yet in the context it was used, it seems the Professor was referring to all Covid-19 patients, whether hospitalized or in the clinic, even though such extrapolation is a deadly sin in clinical trials and in intellectual circles and is definitely not expected at the professorial level. According to **Professor Francois Balloux** (*Computational Systems Biology, Director UCL Genetics Institute*)

> "*The absence of any meaningful benefit of HCQ in the treatment of Covid-19 infections is in line with other comparable clinical trials."*

"Absence of any meaningful benefit" from HCQ is expected in hospitalized patients as far as the average doctor and the rest of the world is concerned. A professor in their field knows more than the average doctor or the media and I am not going to diminish the knowledge base of any British professor to that of a commoner operating under the Gambini influence. These professors should not be making these types of statements as it is of such a rudimentary quality of knowledge as to be degrading mentioning it. Only **Professor Babak Javid** (*Tsinghua University School of Medicine, Infectious Disease Consultant, Cambridge Hospital*) noted that the administration of hydroxychloroquine in hospitalized and severely ill Covid-19 patients and its failure in RECOVERY shouldn't have come as a surprise based on HCQ's mechanism of action. Simply stated, it means HCQ should be given

51

The HCQ Debate, Caxton Opere, MD

early, before hospitalization, and I presume that is what Professor Javid is referring to.

Other professors and doctors wrongfully commending the RECOVERY study include:
Professor Ian Hall, Molecular Medicine *(University of Nottingham)*
Professor Paraston Donyai *(University of Reading)*
Professor Ravi Guptap *(Cambridge University)*
Professor Keith Neil *(University of Nottingham)*
Professor Graham Cooke *(Imperial College)*
Dr. Stephen Griffin Associate Professor School of Medicine *(University of Leeds)*

These professors ignored the patients killed in the name of a hidden Gambini agenda through trusted medical care that turns out to be like the Tuskegee Syphilis experiment.

When I searched for the documents for the actual trial protocols for RECOVERY, I found one on www.recoverytrial.net and the document did not have the dosage of hydroxychloroquine used in the study protocol. As a matter of fact, pages 4 and 5 of the document, as well as pages 24 and 25 for pediatric dosing of the RECOVERY protocol listed hydrocortisone, methylprednisolone, human normal IVIG, azithromycin, convalescent plasma and tocilizumab. No mention was made of hydroxychloroquine in the treatment arm of drugs used in the study. It's as if the investigators finally realized they had used toxic doses of HCQ and intended to wipe off any evidence of the job done. Version 2.0, dated March 21, 2020 listed hydroxychloroquine and by version 7.0 on June 18, 2020 on page 20 of the protocol, there was no longer any HCQ, about the time the investigators announced they were stopping the HCQ arm of the study. Professor Horby, the chief investigator of RECOVERY, should be asked why despite understanding the lethal dose of hydroxychloroquine, allowed such dosing to be used in the study.

Since I couldn't find any traces of the doses of hydroxychloroquine used in RECOVERY on their 30-page protocol, I also did a Google search and on the second try with a really long question I found the dose on the second page of the search at

www.palmerfoundation.com.au

The site stated that

"The HCQ regimen used in the RECOVERY trial was 12 tablets during the first 24 hours (800mg initial dose, 800mg six hours later, 400mg 6 hours later, 400mg 6 hours later), then 400mg every 12 hours for 9 more days. This is 2.4 grams during the first 24 hours, and a cumulative dose of 9.2 grams over 10 days."

If you start HCQ treatment at 5am on Monday morning in the RECOVERY trial this is what it'll look like:

Monday 5am: 800mg
Monday 11am: 800mg
Monday 5pm: 400mg
Monday 11pm: 400mg
Total HCQ dose on Day 1= 2.4g in 18 hours!

According to the RECOVERY protocol, the patient actually gets 2.4g in 18 hours and 2.8g in 24 hour. That's five HCQ doses from 5am on Monday to 5am on Tuesday morning. Also, note that whether it's 2.4g or 2.8g of HCQ in 24 hours, depending on how you see it, this is the total safe 5-day dose recommended by the FDA. On Tuesday morning, you continue again at 5am for every 12 hours for a total of ten days

Tuesday 5am: 400mg
Tuesday 5pm: 400mg
= 800mg daily for 9 more days
= 7.2 grams
Total RECOVERY HCQ dose = 9.6g

So, RECOVERY patients received a total of 9.6g HCQ in ten days, four times the recommended FDA dose. Does it remind you of the Borba et al study? Whether intentionally or not, it seems that the dose of HCQ given in the RECOVERY study was designed to make sure patients don't RECOVER! The chief investigator of RECOVERY, Professor Martin Landray (*Medicine and Epidemiology, Oxford University*), and his deputy chief for the study, Professor Peter Horby (*Emerging Infections and Global Health*) should be asked why they incorporated such toxic if not lethal doses for HCQ in their study design despite sufficient data that such high dosages are not necessary. How many patients died unnecessarily because of this?

53

12
SOLIDARITY

SOLIDARITY is a WHO-sponsored study involving over 100 countries eager to participate in the fight against Covid-19. According to the www.palmerfoundation.com website reviewers of the study, it was difficult for them to find the dosing information on HCQ used in the SOLIDARITY study at the WHO website. The Canadians however had the HCQ dosing used in their SOLIDARITY study:

1. *Lopinavir/ritonavir 400mg/100mg bid for 14 days OR*
2. *Hydroxychloroquine 800mg bid for 1 day then 400mg bid for 10 days OR*
3. *Remdesivir 200mg IV on day 1, followed by 100mg IV daily for 9 days OR*
4. *Optimized supportive care until discharge from hospital or expiration*

All 1-3 above treatment groups also received optimized supportive care. Take note of the HCQ dosing. Within 24 hours, the HCQ group will have received 2.0g, more than the lethal dose of 1.5g chloroquine base.

SOLIDARITY HCQ Regimen:
Day 1: 800mg every 12 hours
Day 2: 400mg every 12 hours x 9 days
= 1.6g (Day 1) + 800mg x 9 (Day 2-10)
= 1.6g + 7.2g
= 8.8g

2g in the first 24 hours

It's important to understand that HCQ is not immediately excreted from the body following ingestion. It accumulates in the body. According to the FDA data, following a single 200mg oral dose of HCQ, its peak concentration is reached in about 3.26 hours, with a half-life of 537 hours (22.4 days). This should help you see what happens when you give even higher doses of HCQ as recorded for the COALITION, Borba et al, RECOVERY AND SOLIDARITY studies. France launched the DisCoVeRy study as its version of SOLIDARITY. DisCoVeRy is an adaptive, randomized, multicenter open 5 parallel arm trial, with a target sample size of 3100 patients with 620 patients per treatment arm in 34 centers. Randomization was 1:1:1:1:1. The population enrolled includes hospitalized patients with Covid-19 and hypoxemia based on clinical and laboratory criteria, with or without respiratory failure. There were 4 intervention arms with or without standard of care (SoC) compared with SoC alone:

1. Remdesivir
2. Lopinavir/Ritonavir
3. Lopinavir/Ritonavir + Beta interferon
4. Hydroxychloroquine
5. Standard of Care alone

Dr. Mondher Toumi and colleagues pointed out some problems with both the SOLIDARITY and DisCoVeRy clinical trials

Problem#1: Protocols Impractical, Disconnected from Reality and Difficult to Implement
In their analysis of both the SOLIDARITY and DisCoVeRy trials, they (Toumi et al) described the clinical trial design as appearing ideal from a methodological perspective but both SOLIDARITY and DisCoVeRy trials appear difficult to implement, impractical and disconnected from the pandemic reality. This is consistent with the failure of both trials to produce helpful conclusions.

Problem #2: Patients Too Far Advanced to benefit from Antiviral Therapy
One of the reasons Toumi et. al gave for their indictment is that the hospitalized population is far too advanced to benefit from antiviral therapy and may benefit more from anti-cytokine release syndrome drugs such as tocilizumab, rituximab or dupilimab and that the protocol was not compliant with Good Clinical Practice (GCP).

Problem #3: Too Many Endpoints Making it Difficult for Practitioners to Participate in Study
Another viewpoint Toumi *et. al* had was that the study had more than 100 endpoints, making it difficult for practitioners to want to participate. The authors of this analytical paper looked at the thoroughness and appropriateness of both studies and had the following to say about the SOLIDARITY TRIAL:

> *"The study provides a very high level design but "the sample size of 50,000 patients resembles more of an all inclusive strategy rather than a conscientiously scientific sample power calculation."*

Solidarity was stopped early due to little or no reduction in mortality. No one knows exactly what the "little" in the study means and it would have been more honorable to at least publish their study findings for other analytical eyes.

Toumi et al described the DisCoVeRy trial design as

> *"lacking pragmatism and failing to take into consideration the behavior of patients."*

No patient will enroll in a placebo arm of a study during a deadly pandemic when a potential treatment is available. This is the exact reason why no physician in their right mind should expect a "gold standard" of prospective, randomized placebo-controlled double-blinded trial for HCQ. It is an unrealistic expectation or an excuse for mediocrity, but a reality of patient behavior. The majority of physicians that have used HCQ used it early in the course of the infection and most report not sixty or seventy percent success but over 95% consistently. The methodological concrete thinker wants randomized placebo-controlled double-blinded trials before accepting that HCQ works but they are probably the same ones that read only the abstract section of the reputable journals without giving any time or thought to the entire article. They forget that when a patient has Covid-19 symptoms and goes to the clinic or hospital, these patients don't want to be in the placebo arm of anything, they just want to be treated with whatever drug is immediately available to avoid death. No one wants to be a placebo guinea pig. If you've seen sick Covid-19 patients in the emergency room and clinic responding to HCQ, you won't insist on double-blinded placebo-controlled randomized gold standard studies of HCQ because you're never going to get such a study during a pandemic. Demanding such a clinical trial is like insisting that the army do double-blinded placebo controlled studies with one half of the soldiers jumping out of the plane without a parachute and the other half using the parachute before you accept that parachutes prevent death when jumping out of a plane. As of this writing, I'm working with a Covid-19 task force in South Texas in a hospital that about two months ago had so many dying Covid-19 patients, the army had to send in a refrigerated vehicle to hold the dead bodies packed in the hallways. So when I hear people, particularly doctors who never had the opportunity to start early treatment with HCQ (aka parachute) insist on RCT's for HCQ's efficacy, I realize we have more than a Covid-19 pandemic on our hands. I could easily have been one of such doctors so I am thankful I am not. I have had the opportunity of helping Covid-19 patients at both the early and intermediate stages of illness, as well as critically ill patients that survived. So hearing from those who do not see patients or face life and death issues with patients and their family members say they need RCT's is laughable but a serious matter. I remember reading an article in which the author argued that the only proof for HCQ's efficacy in SARS-CoV-2 was an in-vitro study showing HCQ's efficacy in tissue culture, reflecting a complete lack of how drug treatment ideas evolve in real life or other clinical trials published in the journals. Such need to be reminded about how penicillin was discovered. This is what happens when doctors without a heart, lacking empathy and compassion, cold, unfeeling, never really taking care of patients still wear the "MD" badge. I think there should be a law amongst doctors that with the exception of retired doctors, if you don't take care of patients for more than 2 years, and are no longer providing direct patient care, you should hold on to a different designation other than MD. You can use Dr. but not MD or perhaps if you're an MD still actively researching, the title should be changed to "MR" meaning medical researcher or medical reader not MD. I think that's one of the major reasons for the ongoing HCQ debate, the fact that some are posing as doctors because they have an MD degree without really knowing what it means to care for patients or deal with the complexities of family, death, poverty, addiction, weakness, hopelessness, uncertainty, fear, normal human irrationality and lack of predictability that "real" doctors do while caring for patients. I could sometimes tell that an author is a medical researcher (MR) rather than a medical doctor (MD) when reading researching journals based on what they called patients enrolled in their clinical trials. It's quite telling!

Problem #4: Toxic HCQ doses Used in Solidarity
SOLIDARITY used toxic HCQ doses totaling 8.8g. Keep in mind that every tablet of HCQ given to the patient is cumulative in effect as the drug has a long half-life. There is not much more to comment further on as the rest of the results were not published and only a press release was made available after the study was cancelled. Of note, the Mehra et al study published in May 2020, in both the *New England Journal of Medicine* and the *Lancet*, was instrumental in temporarily halting the SOLIDARITY study. The Mehra study was however retracted due to lack of important raw data to verify the author's assertions and conclusions. The WHO restarted the study after the protests but halted it again finally in June. Even the French government revoked the use of HCQ based on the retracted-for-lack-of-sufficient-proof Mehra study at the end of May. So if HCQ were effective, a sham study has misled governments to halting the use of a drug that could have potentially saved many lives and prevented an overwhelming of the healthcare system particularly the hospitals in many parts of the world.

57

The HCQ Debate, Caxton Opere, MD

13

HENRY FORD I Study
Arshad S et al. Treatment with HCQ, Azithromycin and Combination in Patients Hospitalized with Covid-19.
Int J Inf Dis. Vol 97:396-403
2541 patients

There were two Covid-19 studies at Henry Ford Hospitals in Detroit. One was a prospective outpatient prophylaxis study using HCQ in high-risk healthcare workers (WHIP study) and the other, a retrospective cohort study of hospitalized patients. For convenience, the inpatient study will from henceforth be called the Henry Ford I study. The latter evaluated all hospitalized patients treated for Covid-19 from March 10, 2020, to May 2, 2020, in order to determine the association between HCQ use and inpatient mortality.

2541 patients with a median hospital length of stay of 6 days, a median age of 64 years with 51% of patients male, 56% African American. Patients received HCQ, HCQ +Azithromycin, or nothing. The primary outcome was in-hospital mortality (death). Even though death is considered to be a crude outcome parameter because many things may have led to it, it still may be a decent measure since severe Covid-19 is short term and benefits of treatment or lack thereof are equally measurable as short-term events and the majority of people that die from Covid-19 wouldn't have died suddenly all other things being equal. So unlike what we evaluate following a heart attack where we're interested in after discharge mortality say in 30 days or a year, for Covid-19, it's usually a shorter period to anticipate the death impact. 82% of the patients received HCQ within 24 hours and 91% received HCQ within 48 hours of the study and primary outcome was in-hospital mortality.

Overall mortality was 18.1% with respiratory failure being the primary cause of death in 88% of these deaths and no patient had Torsades de pointes.

Predictors of death in the study were:
Age 65 or older HR 2.6 (1.9-3.3)
White Race HR 1.7 (1.4-2.1)

Hypoxia on admission HR 1.5 (1.1-2.1)
Ventilator use HR 2.2 (1.4-3.3)

Treatment with HCQ alone provided a 66% hazard ratio reduction and treatment with the combination of HCQ and azithromycin provided a 71% hazard ratio reduction. The study showed that HCQ did help in reducing death in hospitalized patients. Some critics attacked this study and it's probably because it showed benefit for HCQ and the Gambini factor was hard at work. Things got so bad that the Vice President of Medical Affairs of the Henry Ford Hospital System with another high ranking hospital administrator had to write a letter to the public about the idiocy of such attacks and promised to no longer share their information with the public. In that manner we may never know the outcome of the second outpatient WHIP study since Henry Ford officials are fully aware that the Gambini people will come after them with prongs and spears. As long as they do not attempt to misguide clinicians or provided toxic doses of treatment, pandemic studies on Covid-19 treatment cannot be perfect.

The HCQ Debate, Caxton Opere, MD

14

NYU, Carlucci P et al, 2020.
Hydroxychloroquine and azithromycin plus zinc vs. Hydroxychloroquine and azithromycin alone: Outcomes in hospitalized Covid-19 patients Observational study. 922 patients

The last inpatient clinical trial we will look at before examining some outpatient studies is actually a transitional study in the sense that it provides not only a new paradigm of inpatient management but also an explanation of a critical element of outpatient Covid-19 management. Most of the public is already aware of the use of zinc in Covid-19. While many doctors with information from half-baked poorly designed, executed or reported studies are caught in the middle of nowhere in terms of knowing how to treat Covid-19 patients in the absence of definitive treatments, they forget the reason for their confusion is right before their eyes; poorly designed studies, some intended to kill patients. We now have doctors passively watching their patients die while still arguing that there are no randomized placebo-controlled double-blinded studies to prove the efficacy of HCQ. So this study is at least helpful in terms of pointing to an inexpensive direction for managing Covid-19 patients. While paid Gambini stooges may attack the study, you ought to be familiar with how Covid-19 infection should be safely and sanely managed.

Setting was the NYU Langone Hospital system in New York. This is an observational study and the authors gracefully stated that it is not a clinical trial. Dignified! Particularly when compared with the withdrawn May 22, 2020 Lancet and May 1, 2020 NEJM articles that were withdrawn after discovering that the questionable data the authors used may have been fabricated. So think about it for minute. Why would professors and eminent physicians want to use fabricated data? Is Boris or Dr. Gambini responsible for such behavior? Even the mere thought of fabricating such data and the WHO basing their decision to cancel their own HCQ trials as a result of these journals authored by the same physicians makes you think of Dr. Gambini. Once the semi-scandal was discovered, WHO quickly retracted and restarted their trials. That makes me wonder but I won't share any thoughts or ideas.

Treatment Regimen at NYU Langone Hospital
HCQ 400mg once then

HCQ 200mg twice daily x 4 days
Azithromycin 500mg daily x 5 days
Zinc sulfate capsule 220mg twice daily x 5 days (220mg capsule contained 50mg elemental zinc)

Patients in the two treatment arms
HCQ +AZi+Zinc Sulfate; N = 411
HCQ+ Azi; N = 521

This study may be a can opener for worms that pharmaceutical companies are afraid the world might discover. They think the world and even doctors are blind but the world has already woken up, they just don't know where the rest of the information to help complete the picture puzzle is located, at least not just yet! I'm going to share with you some of these once we get past the outpatient studies. This NYU study is the first study reporting the use of hydroxycholoroquine and zinc in hospitalized Covid-19 patients. It doesn't boast of being a clinical trial and is an observational study that provides the first in vivo evidence that zinc sulfate in combination with hydroxchloroquine can be an effective therapeutic strategy for hospitalized Covid-19 patients, a far cry from many of the previous studies mentioned earlier in this book.

Data collection via electronic medical records of patients admitted rom March 2 to April 5, 2020. Addition of zinc sulfate did not impact length of hospitalization, duration of ventilation or ICU stay. The study also underwent univariate analyses, that is, data analysis in which a single variable is examined to find a pattern without trying to establish cause or relationships. When this univariate analysis was done, zinc sulfate

1. Increased the frequency of patients being discharged home; OR 1.53, 95% CI 1.12-2.09
2. Decreased the need for mechanical ventilation
3. Decreased admission to the ICU
4. Decreased the risk of death or transfer to hospice (futility) OR 0.449, 95% CI 0.271-0.744

The authors reported that the main findings of the study were
1. After adjusting for the timing of zinc therapy, the addition of zinc sulfate to hydroxychloroquine and azithromycin was associated with a decrease in mortality but this association was not significant in patients treated in the ICU.
2. There was a potential synergistic therapeutic advantage of combining HCQ with zinc sulfate if used early in presentation

The HCQ Debate, Caxton Opere, MD

"In bivariate logistic regression analysis, the addition of zinc sulfate was associated with decreased mortality or transition to hospice (OR 0.511, 95% CI 0.359-0.726)

decreased need for ICU (OR 0.545, 95% CI 0.362-0.821

decreased need for invasive ventilation (OR 0.562, 95% CI 0.354-0.891.

However after excluding all non-critically ill patients admitted to the ICU, zinc sulfate was no longer found to be associated with decreased mortality. So what role dose zinc play in Covid-19 infection? The answer, found in chapter 30, will surprise you.

15

HCQ: What All Doctors Should Know

Hydroxychloroquine is not the drug Americans are told it is. It is a very good drug, not a very dangerous one. Before getting deeper into the zinc factor and looking at outpatient studies on hydroxchloroquine that are already published, it's important to emphasize a few points about hydroxchloroquine, and its immediate cousin, chloroquine phosphate. Both are used in the treatment of malaria as long as it is not chloroquine-resistant malaria. HCQ is also used in treating systemic lupus as well as rheumatoid arthritis. It has a multiple number of side effects ranging from ocular toxicity, gastrointestinal effects, cardiac arrhythmias, hypotension, dizziness, myopathy, hypoglycemia, hypokalemia and extrapyramidal symptoms. Many actively practicing physicians all over the world attest to the efficacy of HCQ in Covid-19 patients, particularly in non-hospitalized patients. Perhaps because of politics, HCQ has been discredited in the United States, probably to the detriment of its own people. That may explain why the US currently has the highest incidence of infection and Covid-19 deaths to date. Refusal to acknowledge what works even if it's not the perfect drug, and for trusted authorities to generate double-speak that in turn leads to unnecessary controversies about effective infection control methods such as the use of masks have contributed to these high Covid-19 numbers in the United States. Thanks to some Government officials, some people in the United States don't know if they should be wearing a mask to protect themselves or others.

GENERAL MECHANISM OF ACTION OF HCQ
Once inside the cell, HCQ increases endosomal pH, thereby impairing cellular enzyme processes and protein synthesis. It also impairs viral receptor gylcosylation. HCQ inhibits toll-like-receptor signaling, and decreases production of cytokines especially IL-1 and IL-6 (*Savarion et al. Lancet Infect Dis. 2003;3(11):722-727*). It also has been shown to protect from thrombovascular events in SLE patients. (*Arthritis Rheum. 2010; 62(3):863-868*).

COVID-19 SPECIFIC MECHANISMS OF ACTION

The spike protein of the SARS-CoV-2 virus is made up of two subunits, S1 and S2. The S1 subunit allows attachment to the ACE-2 receptor on

The HCQ Debate, Caxton Opere, MD

the type II pneumocyte in the lungs of the host. The type II pneumocyte is responsible for producing surfactant and lowering surface tension in the alveoli. The S2 subunit allows fusion of the virus with the host cell membrane. Once the virus fuses with the host cell membrane, an inward envelope is formed called an endosome. The viral genetic material RNA stays inside this endosome until it receives a signal to release the genetic material of the virus. One of the signals that triggers the endosome to release the viral genetic material is a drop in the pH inside the endosome (envelope). HCQ prevents this drop in pH by raising the pH in the environment. Remember that chloroquine is a weak base and so it increases the pH inside the cell thereby eliminating the acidic environment needed for the release of the genetic material of the virus. This automatically means that HCQ can hinder virus multiplication if it is given early, before the virus captures the manufacturing plant for virus replication inside the host cell. This is a sound scientific process that has been established previously about how HCQ can prevent multiplication of the SARS-CoV-2 virus when given early.

The second established scientific mechanism by which HCQ attacks the SARS-CoV-2 virus is by preventing the virus from attaching to the receptors in the lungs. Before SARS-CoV-2 can attach and lock firmly to the ACE-2 receptor on the type II pneumocyte in the lungs, its spike protein must first be activated by transmembrane protease serine 2 (TMPS2). This activation requires a chemical process called glycosylation. Glycosylation is the addition of a sugar molecule to a chemical. HCQ prevents the glycosylation step that allows the spike protein to attach to the ACE-2 receptor. It's funny to think of it this way but you can say that the greedy virus needs some sugar and HCQ will not let it get the sugar. This should also help you remember one of the side effects of HCQ, hypoglycemia.

It's important to understand the science behind the use of HCQ in Covid-19 infection. Forget the drama and the poorly conceived research data. Focus on possibilities. Ask the right questions. You might find it difficult if you have methodically built up hatred for the world's number one personality attached to HCQ based on the Cheyenko Method, President Donald Trump. You'll need to purge yourself of that hatred and cognitive bias, particularly if you're in the medical field or have enough wisdom that people might seek your opinion on Covid-19 issues. Otherwise you may mislead people to their death or detriment. Unfortunately, many have died unnecessarily because they were denied therapy with HCQ and Gambini has sent out many reporters and journalists to fuel the propaganda about HCQ's toxicity and lack of efficacy even though the scientific evidence in favor of HCQ is there as is the opportunity to get HCQ. If you want to give HCQ, you should give it before the patient gets really sick as to require hospitalization, and before they became critically ill. If you want to know more about many of the HCQ trials in one place visit I do recommend https://hcqtrial.com.

There, you'll find a host of studies summarized on HCQ and a brief analysis with study classifications into early or late use, and whether HCQ was given as pre-exposure or post exposure prophylaxis. There were 103 in vivo studies of HCQ in Covid-19; 62 were for late treatment, 24 were for early treatment, 3 were post-exposure prophylaxis, 14 pre-exposure prophylaxis studies, with positive rates of HCQ efficacy of 63%, 100%, 100% and 89% respectively. Epidemiologists really went out to slice the owners of this website because they made a technical christening blunder, calling their report a study trial. and using terminology meant only for actual studies. For example, they stated that since governments in some countries decided not to use HCQ/CQ while others decided to do so, those countries that chose HCQ/CQ were randomized to the treatment group while those that did not choose HCQ/CQ were automatically randomized to the non-treatment group. Christening error, misuse of randomization, and they almost got burnt at the stake. If you really don't want patients to die from Covid-19 and want to do something about the pandemic you will need objective information about HCQ, the only drug that is effective in early Covid-19 infection besides the Ivermectin/doxycycline combo. I recommend you visit the website above in spite of what has been said about them as you will see a true collation of over 100 studies and gather the knowledge you need to cut through the maze of confusion from journalistic terrorism. They have links that can take you directly to the original study paper or abstract. Journalistic because they are the ones propagating most of the false information even though their training enables them to investigate and uncover all the information you have read so far in this book. Terrorism, because too many patients have died because of the deliberate one-sided information propagated by journalists. This behavior has cost over a million deaths and is truly the greatest act of terrorism of our time. The mere fact that this website exists while journalists keep spreading misinformation about the lack of efficacy of HCQ for Covid-19 is a sure sign they've been bought and under the influence of the Cheyenko program. Epidemiologists, which I am not, hate the website and perhaps the venom displayed against the authors of the website reflects one of the issues of this pandemic, an air of

65

The HCQ Debate, Caxton Opere, MD

superiority based on their training without any indication that they care about the shoddily designed lethally dosed programs.

Avoid websites that appear to provide information on Covid-19 but are not only biased in their relentless anti-HCQ campaigns, they attack doctors getting results but do not offer actual treatment strategies for those seeking such information.

Table showing multiple staging and clinical features of Covid-19

4 Stages of Infection	Biologic Onset	Early Infection	Usual stage diagnosis	Outcome = Resolved or IV, V or VI		
Diagnosis	Impossible	Hard	Easiest	Easy	-	-
Clinical Stage	Asymptomatic	Mild	Moderate	Severe	Critical	Dead
Numeric Staging	I	II	III	IV	V	VI
*O2 Sat %	100%	98	96	94	92	
Alveoli						
**Tx Type	Pre Exposure	Postexposure	Early	Late	Very Late	Too Late
***EUA/FDA	No	No	No	Yes	Yes	-
HCQ Efficacy	89%	100%	100%	63%		

*.O2 Saturation is the percentage from the baseline. So if the patient had a baseline of 96% for example and their O2 saturation now drops to 92%, he or she is now stage III Covid-19 not critical.
**. Tx type = Treatment type. The first category in this row is called pre-exposure as disease is undetectable. Note that this group also includes

rheumatology patients already on HCQ for either rheumatoid arthritis (RA) or lupus.

***EUA/FDA**. The FDA's EUA for HCQ recommends it be given when it has negligible or zero effect. It would be interesting to know who drew up this EUA.

According to hcqtrials.com,

> *"Many countries either adopted or declined early treatment with HCQ, effectively forming a large trial with 1.8 billion people in the treatment group and 663 million in the control group. As of September 20, 2020, an average of 70.1/million people in the treatment group have died, and 477.2 per million in the control group, relative risk 0.147. After adjustments, treatment and control, deaths became 146.8 per million and 715.0 per million, relative risk 0.2 (in the treatment and control groups respectively). The probability of an equal or lower relative risk occurring from random group assignments is 0.015. (p=0.015). The treatment group (HCQ) has a 73.9% lower death rate."*

Are you surprised Gambini's journalists haven't mentioned this?

When you look at the EUA for HCQ, it has no scientific basis, and much of the so-called scientific evidence against the use of HCQ in outpatients is prefabricated, cognitively biased, and based on dangerously executed studies in hospitalized patients that have been so publicized they drown out the use of HCQ and monger fear in American physicians. On June 15, 2020, Denise M. Hinton, the FDA's Chief Scientist, addressed a letter to Dr. Gary Disbrow, Deputy Assistant Secretary of the US Department of Health and Human Services Biomedical Advanced Research and Development Authority (BARDA) division, granting Dr. Disbrow's request to revoke the EUA for HCQ. Not one single study was cited in Denise Hinton's letter regarding the research that enabled him to arrive at a reasonable conclusion regarding HCQ's lack of efficacy in early Covid-19 infection. Any physician, healthcare professional or concerned and critically thinking individual who understands science and the mechanism of action of HCQ in Covid-19, will immediately see that the EUA itself was misleading in its indication for use of HCQ. As I mentioned multiple times in *COVID-19: Physician Treatment Strategies*, HCQ should be given early not at the advanced stages of Covid-19 infection. To wait till the patient becomes hypoxic or needs hospitalization means you have waited too late. As you can see from the

67

mechanisms of action of HCQ outlined above in the previous paragraphs, it is impossible to imagine that a bunch of government scientists would concoct an EUA for use of HCQ when it will be least effective. The question I have is how is it possible that a United States government official with many years of experience and perhaps brilliance will allow such an EUA to be passed? Besides this, the administration of HCQ to hospitalized patients makes absolutely no sense medically (pharmacologically and pathologically), or epidemiologically.

Figure. 1. Declining efficacy of HCQ with time. *(Bouleware et al, 2020)*

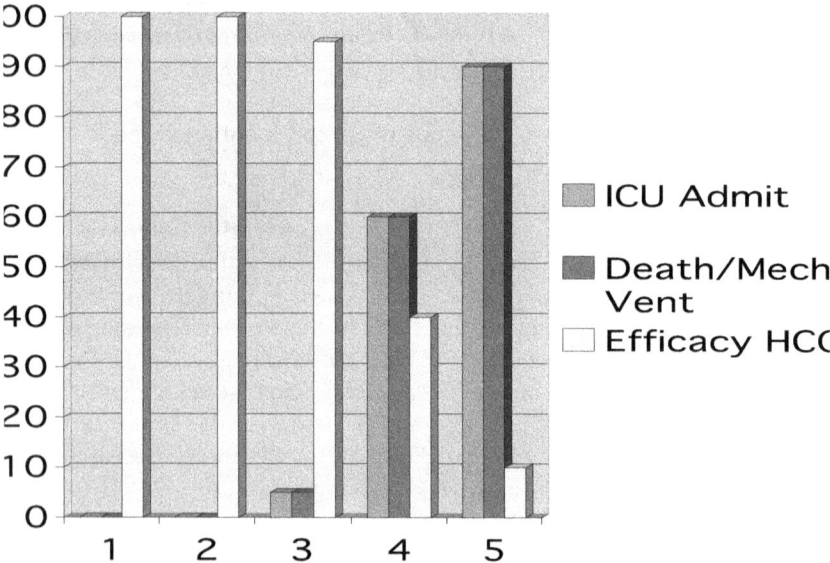

Pharmacologically, the FDA's hydroxychloroquine EUA completely ignored the stages at which the immunomodulatory and viral replication blocking benefits of HCQ would be maximized, that is, early during the infection. Pathologically, the viral replication triggers immunological and biochemical reactions to go completely haywire and HCQ cannot be expected to control such poorly understood mechanisms when they occur that late in the disease. There are also some other complex processes involved in the Covid-19 disease process. For example, it is only recently that Bradykinin is thought to play a role in what was thought to be a cytokine storm. Epidemiologically, the EUA ignores the majority of those still at risk of getting infected and are most likely to benefit the most from getting HCQ early following exposure. Had the EUA been thoughtfully not just rapidly designed, perhaps those designing it, assuming they do not work for Dr. Gambini, would have seen that the most logical place for HCQ administration of HCQ was in the 80% with mild disease following exposure and the other 10 to 15 percent with moderate symptoms with no clear indication for hospitalization, and not the 5 percent critically ill and hospitalized patients. The EUA was basically turned upside down.

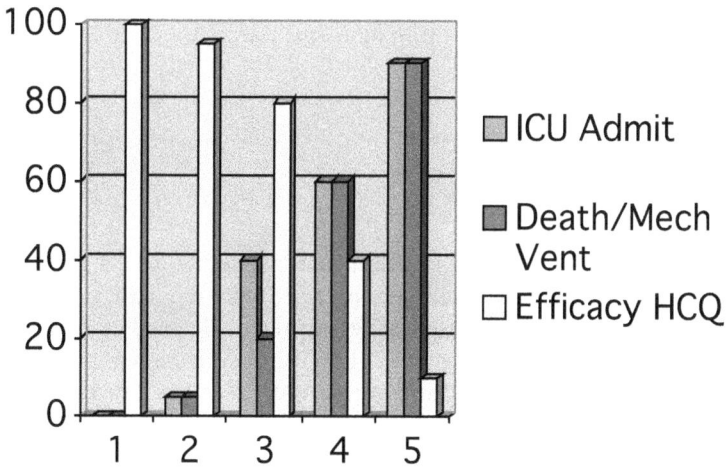

STAGE 4, the stage at which there is a precipitous drop in HCQ efficacy in Covid-19, is where the revoked EUA by the US FDA recommended that HCQ be started. This is not the best place to start HCQ but I don't see any of our clinical trial experts denounce this recommendation and wonder why. Notice how risk of ICU admission and death rise with time and how efficacy of HCQ declines with time. Even then, some studies still show efficacy with HCQ with or without zinc or azithromycin in hospitalized patients.

The HCQ Debate, Caxton Opere, MD

As you can see from the above chart, the FDA's revoked EUA for HCQ recommended that HCQ only be given to hospitalized patients at stage IV Covid-19. This is at a time when the patients are severely ill, hospitalized, at 94% or less from their baseline oxygen saturation and with a 60% chance of getting admitted to the intensive care unit, (ICU), ending on mechanical ventilation for respiratory failure, or dying from Covid-19. This is also the time when the efficacy of HCQ in Cvid-19 drops precipitously. The WHO said HCQ is not recommended in Covid-19, but there's a reason the head of the WHO is not a doctor capable of making clinical decisions. Many HCQ detractors have designed their toxic studies to drive home their point, killing or maiming many innocent, and intending to kill millions more in their quest to prove that "HCQ is ineffective". Most of the studies showing lack of efficacy of HCQ were in advanced disease in hospitalized patients and the media's often cited studies of lack of efficacy of HCQ in outpatients draw their wisdom from studies like the Brazilian and Bouleware et al studies.

Indications for Use of HCQ
Infections. Rheumatologic disorders. Off-label use in porphyria uses as 200mg twice a week.

Malaria.
HCQ increases the pH of the acidic food vacuoles of the erythrocytic forms of the *Plasmodium* parasite, and diminishing vesicle function as well as reproduction of the parasite asexually (*Kaur et al 2010*). It also inhibits parasite growth by interfering with the conversion of toxic heme resulting from the plasmodium ingesting hemoglobin to the non-toxic hemozoin. (*Pandey et al, 2003*)

RA
Increases the pH in the lysosomes of antigen presenting cells, blocking toll-like receptors on dendritic cells and reducing the activation of the cells. HCQ stabilizes the lysosomal membranes of white blood cells thereby preventing the release of enzymes that breakdown cartilage such as collagenase and protease.

Porphyria
HCQ is used off-label in porphyria.

Retinopathy
As long as patients receive a daily dose of less than 5mg/kg for less than 10 years, the incidence of retinopathy was relatively low at 2%. The risk

went up to 20% for those patients who had taken HCQ for over 20 years. *(Wolfe & Marmor, 2010; Melles & Marmor 2014)*. No clinician ever talks about retinopathy for acute short-term use of HCQ, except in cases of acute poisoning. There are some online sites that provide more details about HCQ ocular toxicity but the cumulative dose leading to retinopathy is at least 5 years and more likely to be ten years. Mentioning retinopathy in acute use of HCQ over a 7-day period is simply implanting wrong ideas in the minds of doctors unfamiliar with the use of HCQ.

Proposed Future Indications for HCQ
Chemotherapy. Viral infections.

HCQ has a role, a very significant one, in the management of Covid-19 infections. Denying it that role has cost the United States billions if not trillions in economic losses. We seem surprised that the USA continues to have the highest number of Covid-19 cases and deaths. While many countries are using HCQ, and have avoided the political drama Americans have stubbornly attached to HCQ because they hate their President, other countries, even poor ones, are doing what they need to do to lower their incidence of new cases. Americans are fighting the wrong Covid-19 battle by attacking doctors prescribing HCQ and getting excellent results. And the press is no less guilty of the blood of the innocent. A self-inflicted problem indeed! You won't wear a mask, you won't take HCQ and you won't research to find out what other countries are doing to control Covid-19 infection. Common sense tells you that the staff inside the hospital are not getting infected in their extremely high risk environments simply because the hospital staff are wearing masks and face-shields and those involved with direct patient care on Covid-19 floors are the only ones wearing extra personal protective equipment (PPE) when needed. For those anti-maskers, it's unlikely that they ever sat down to think about why most hospital staff are not getting Covid-19 positive! It's the mask, and the silent HCQ users! I suppose that the Gambini group will be satisfied as long as these HCQ users and prescribers stay silent long enough for them to carry out any agenda they have in mind.

The HCQ Debate, Caxton Opere, MD

16

ACUTE TOXICITY OF HCQ AND CQ

Shortly after the world learnt about the potential use of chloroquine and hydroxychloroquine in SARS-CoV-2 infection in early 2020, some "civilians" took matters into their own hands. While in the previous decades the WHO reported only about 35 reports of fatal acute chloroquine poisoning, cases of chloroquine and hydroxychloroquine overdose, began to appear in the news and in medical journals. It's important to understand what happens with an overdose of chloroquine or hydroxychloroquine. The FDA data on HCQ (Plaquenil®) states that following ingestion of a 200mg dose of hydroxychloroquine, a mean peak blood concentration of 129.6ng/mL is reached in 3.26 hours. With the same dose, a peak plasma concentration of 50.3ng/mL is reached at 3.76 hours. Blood and plasma concentrations differ for HCQ as you can see. At the daily doses recommended in the FDA's EUA, usual side effects are often transient and include, nausea, dizziness, anorexia, abdominal pain or discomfort, generalized itching, tingling. Even rarer are the abnormal involuntary movements that may include facial tics, involuntary tongue protrusions, excessive salivation, or neck muscle spasms. The involuntary movements can occur with a single dose of hydroxychloroquine and has been reported in children.

There are two main groups of patients presenting to a hospital with acute chloroquine poisoning; young children in whom overdose is usually accidental, and older adults due to suicidal intent *(Weniger, 1979)*. Now thanks to fundamental violations in human experimentation regulations, a third previously unheard of category in six decades now exists, doctor-induced acute chloroquine poisoning, as well as a fourth, self-induced overdose without suicidal intent in adults. The latter refer to adults who were swallowing self-prescribed large doses of chloroquine and hydroxychloroquine for fear of getting or dying from Covid-19. Chronic toxicity can occur in rheumatologic patients on hydroxychloroquine for lupus or rheumatoid arthritis and this chronic toxicity leads to cardiomyopathy, extrapyramidal effects, hearing loss, ringing in the ears, gait disturbance as well as retinopathy and blindness. Acute toxicity is the one that most physicians and family member need to be aware of as should all investigators using HCQ in Covid-19 or other disorders.

When you look at the studies, those with the lowest total doses of 2 to 2.4g of HCQ seemed to have had the best outcomes, with the exception of Dr. Didier Raoult's 6g total. HCQ is metabolized by the liver and excreted in the urine. When the patient is critically ill and on multiple medications, the liver detoxification process can be overwhelmed even from normal doses of HCQ. In addition, HCQ by itself can cause acute liver injury. Therefore giving ridiculously high or toxic doses of HCQ to sick hospitalized patients is tantamount to killing the patient. It's however possible that as part of the Gambini plan, the decision to overwhelm the liver using toxic doses of HCQ was seen as another subtle opportunity to destroy HCQ's reputation. To give you a clearer understanding of the toxicity risk with HCQ when poorly administered as done in many of the clinical trials mentioned earlier, there was a special 1979 WHO report (WHO/MAL/79.906) prepared by a WHO consultant, H. Weniger. The report, titled *Review of Side Effects and Toxicity of Chloroquine*, made some salient points about CQ toxicity:

1. A 200mg dose of hydroxychloroquine contains 155mg chloroquine base
2. A 250mg dose of chloroquine phosphate contains 150mg chloroquine base
3. A single dose of 300mg chloroquine was fatal in a 3-year old
4. Chloroquine has a narrow therapeutic margin in children
5. Between 1955 and 1978, there were 335 cases of acute chloroquine poisoning in adults resulting in 135 deaths.
6. A single dose of 1.5g to 2.0g of chloroquine may be fatal
7. Cardiac muscle retains more chloroquine than any other muscle (*Armand et al., 1971*)

A 200mg tablet of hydroxychloroquine contains 155mg chloroquine base. To calculate how much chloroquine base you have given to a patient, multiply the hydroxychloroquine sulfate (HCQ) dose given by .775 or the chloroquine phosphate dose by 0.6. So if you gave 800mg of HCQ you have given 620mg of chloroquine base and if you give 600mg of chloroquine phosphate, you have given a total of 360mg chloroquine base. HCQ is 40% less toxic than CQ. Note that there is a difference between whole blood concentrations of chloroquine and plasma concentrations. For a given dose of HCQ, peak blood concentration of chloroquine is usually about 2.57 that in plasma after almost 4 hours.

As opposed to providing guidance to researchers using highly toxic or lethal doses of HCQ or CQ in clinical trials, Watson et al, in an eLife article, reassured us that the toxic or lethal doses in trials like

The HCQ Debate, Caxton Opere, MD

SOLIDARITY or RECOVERY were not really that lethal. *(Watson et al, eLife 2020;9:e58631)*. The authors (Watson et al, 2020) posit that most high dose regimens used in Covid-19 trials are unlikely to cause serious cardiovascular toxicity. This is a very contradictory statement. Most clinical trials on Covid-19 that were attacked as lacking efficacy or associated with HCQ-induced cardiac toxicity and mortality did not use highly toxic doses of HCQ. For example mean daily dose of hydroxychloroquine in Dr. Mehra's retracted Lancet paper was a mean of 596mg daily for 4.2 days or a total of 2.5g, a number still very close to the FDA's revoked hydroxychloroquine EUA total dose of 2.4g HCQ. *Watson et al* used mathematical models to make clinical judgments without considering the clinical condition of sick Covid-19 patients. They seem to have forgotten that their model is based on physically healthy patients taking an overdose of HCQ and want to apply their findings to critically ill Covid-19 patients experiencing respiratory or multi-organ failure. Watson and colleagues analyzed EKG's from healthy French volunteers and compared these EKG's with those from French self-poisoning patients to generate a model. The problem with models is that they can be wrong and in this case, the model was not between sick patient and sick patients but between sick patients and physically healthy patients. Watson tells us that the 600mg twice daily dosing in the study by Borba et al was not lethal but their models were based on healthy patients not critically ill hypoxic patients dying from Covid-19 infection. Even Borba et al admit their HCQ doses were cardiotoxic. Is there a Gambini factor at work here? The models Watson and his colleagues used may not be useful in Covid-19 patients getting lethal doses of HCQ. Based on the Watson model, Borba et al should not even have stopped their clinical trial. But that trial was stopped because of the cardiac toxicity that the Watson model could not predict. One good thing about the Watson paper is that they provide two concrete numbers that could be used as baselines. One of them is that a whole *blood concentration of 13.5μmol/L chloroquine was associated with 1% mortality in* chloroquine self-poisoning cases. That number will probably be much lower for sicker Covid-19 patients with already compromised organs and systems. Less would be required to kill them. Nevertheless it's still a number and something to work from, until you decide to do your own math.

Based on the FDA information on Plaquenil®, a 200mg dose of hydroxychloroquine will reach a peak blood level of 129.6ng/ml in 3.26 hours. Using that simple formula to help us find our way around chloroquine toxicity, let's look at the number Watson et al gave in a different light.

We will assume first order kinetics, that is, what you ingest is directly proportional to the rise in blood levels. In acute poisoning it will often be higher than this calculation but we'll stick to it in order to help us better understand Watson et al's paper and HCQ poisoning. According to the WHO's basic analytical toxicology conversion tool,

$$Chloroquine\ mg/L = \mu mol/L \times 0.32$$
$$Chloroquine\ \mu mol/L = 3.13 \times mg/L$$

So if a blood concentration of 13.5μmol/L is associated with a 1% mortality following self-poisoning, we need to know how many mg of chloroquine base will produce a chloroquine blood level of 13.5μmol/L. To do that we must first convert 13.5μmol/L chloroquine to ng/ml and then determine how many tablets of CQ will give us a blood level of 13.5 μmol/L. Since we know that one 200mg tablet of HCQ produces a blood level of 129.6ng/ml, we can calculate how many pills of HCQ will produce a chloroquine blood level of 13.5μmol/L.

$$13.5\ \mu mol/L\ chloroquine = 13.5 \times 0.32 mg/L = 4.32 mg/L$$
$$4.32 mg/L = 4.32 \mu g\ /ml = 4320 ng/ml$$

So the lethal dose estimated by Dr. Watson's dose is a chloroquine blood level of 4320ng/ml. That would be equal to 4320/129.6 tablets or 33.3 tablets. 33.3 tablets each containing 200mg HCQ is 6.6g of hydroxychloroquine. Remember that the lethal dose of chloroquine according to the WHO is 1.5g. This means that the Watson threshold is 4.4 times higher than the lethal threshold of 1.5g. Little wonder then that Watson and colleagues think the doses given to patients in RECOVERY and other studies are acceptable when in fact they are deadly. That's the problem that arises when a person chooses computerized models rather than analyze data from real patients. Or is there a Gambini factor at work?

The Watson study also revealed that a *QRS duration > 150ms independently predicts mortality in chloroquine self-poisoning*.

ACUTE HCQ POISONING

> *Dr. Rebecca Kruisselbrink and Dr. Zaki Hmen reported the case of a 23-year old female with a history of rheumatoid arthritis on 200mg*

The HCQ Debate, Caxton Opere, MD

daily of HCQ who presented to the hospital after ingesting 8g of HCQ. She remained completely alert and oriented but was in profound shock with a blood pressure of 60/40, severe hypokalemia of 2.1 and a metabolic acidosis with a pH of 7.16. She was intubated, started on vasopressors, bicarbonate, potassium replacement and other supportive care. She recovered completely in 48 hours. (Am J Respir Crit Care Med 181; 2010:A6080).

So it's not just the lethal dose but how quickly the medical team can reach a diagnosis and start immediate treatment that determines the outcomes in HCQ poisoning. If instead, it's the medical team loading the patient with toxic doses of HCQ when the patient is already critically ill with multi-organ malfunction or failure, then we have a serious ethical problem on our hands.

Patients with acute HCQ toxicity can present with respiratory depression, headache, hearing loss, tinnitus, vestibular dysfunction, intractable hypoglycemia, severe intractable hypotension, myopathy, intractable hypokalemia, cardiac arrhythmias, prolonged conduction intervals (PR, QRS, QT), Torsades de pointes, cardiovascular collapse, pulmonary edema and syncope. Hearing loss is due to potassium channel inhibition on outer cochlear hair cells. One of the best articles on acute HCQ and CQ toxicity can be found as part of the Elsevier Public Health Emergency Collection, *Acute Chloroquine and Hydroxychloroquine toxicity: A Review for Emergency Clinicians.* **(Porta, Bornstein, & Coye et al. Am J Emerg Med. 2020. Jul 19.)** Resuscitation as well as poison control principles must be immediately executed in patients suspected of acute CQ or HCQ poisoning. **Rapid decontamination, intravenous fluids, activated charcoal, IV thiamine, intravenous glucose** boluses and infusions, **vasopressor** support, cardiac monitoring, frequent blood sugar checks, and if necessary **endotracheal intubation** must all be considered and executed as deemed necessary by the clinician. Do not induce vomiting. **Diazepam** in doses of 2mg/kg IV given over 30 minutes can be used to manage hypotension and dysrhythmia. The use of diazepam in hypotension might seem like a paradox and has generated some controversy **(Yanturali S, Resuscitation. Volume 63, issue 3 p347-348. December 1, 2004)** but it has been found useful.

According to an article posted on April 14, 2020 on the American College of Toxicology website, the mechanism of action of diazepam in HCQ overdose and subsequent cardiotoxicity remains unclear and could be due to (a) an electrophysiologic effect, (b) an anticonvulsant effect (c) a pharmacokinetic interaction between CQ and diazepam (d) an antidysrhythmic effect by an electrophysiologic action inverse to CQ's effect (e) decrease in CQ-induced vasodilation. Diazepam should be given only when high doses are suspected or confirmed and one study of moderate ingestion (>2g but <4g) did not show a difference in outcomes in patients receiving diazepam. (Clemessy et al. 1996).

For nausea and vomiting, **meclizine** and **metoclopramide** are considered safer due to the QT prolongation associated with ondasetron and phenothiazines. Of utmost importance is that time is of the essence in acute chloroquine overdose because HCQ not only peaks in the blood in about 3.26 hours after ingestion, its average half-life is weeks not hours. (40 days) and it is highly protein bound making dialysis a futile exercise. **Poison control center** should be involved whenever there is suspected acute HCQ or CQ poisoning. **Replace potassium.** Hypokalemia is directly proportional to the degree of poisoning but giving high doses of potassium to replace the hypokalemia can result in rebound severe hyperkalemia as toxicity improves with treatment and with time. Refractory hypoglycemia with glucose levels lower than 50mg/dl should be treated with 50μg of **octreotide** subcutaneously and **glucose infusions**. **Magnesium sulfate** should be given in Torsades des pointes but is not routinely recommended in QT prolongation as per Porta et al. Saline boluses for hypotension and epinephrine with norepinephrine can be given as needed. Care should be taken when giving epinephrine infusions to ensure hypokalemia is not worsened. **Epinephrine** was started at an infusion dose of .25μg/kg/minute by porta et al but I will err on the .15ug/kg/minute side and titrated up. Check blood levels of potassium regularly. Sodium channel blockade can be managed with hypertonic saline (3% NaCl), **sodium bicarbonate** or sodium acetate. Hypertonic saline is infused at 2-4mEq/kg, sodium acetate at 1mEq/kg over 15 minutes and sodium bicarbonate as a bolus of 1-2mEq/kg. Sodium bicarbonate can be repeated as necessary while hoping for termination of any arrhythmia or conduction defects. Whenever these sodium infusions are administered, **always check potassium levels for hypokalemia** which could be worsened from typical cationic displacement of potassium by the infused sodium. **Hemodialysis is ineffective** in HCQ/CQ toxicity due to the high protein binding. Approximately 50% of CQ is excreted by the kidneys and not only can HCQ cause acute renal failure, preexisting renal failure can reduce excretion of HCQ and in turn increase the risk of renal HCQ toxicity. ECMO and hyperbaric oxygen may also be helpful and **hyperbaric oxygen** was reported to help in reversal of visual loss.

The HCQ Debate, Caxton Opere, MD

The highest toxic ingested dose of HCQ reported so far was 22g *(Yanturi et al. Acta Anaesthesiol. Scand 2004; 48: 379-381)*, and the patient developed hypotension, pulseless ventricular tachycardia and mild hypokalemia. She was managed with dopamine, saline boluses, activated charcoal, lidocaine, magnesium sulfate and defibrillation and she survived. No value has been found for serum alkalinization. *(Marquardt & Albertson. Am J Emerg Med 2001;19:420-424).*

17

A Tale of Two Doctors!

Dr. Axel (Dr. A), a Columbia PreMed/Harvard Med School graduate, is a busy internist in private practice. He breezes through medical journals once a week and subscribes to the reputable NEJM, Annals of Internal Medicine, as well as one office practice publication. When he has time he browses through the front cover of the journal for an interesting topic. If he finds one, he looks at the abstract section on the first page of the paper, reads the conclusion, and moves on to the next article. He believes he is well informed on what's going in the medical world and his medical news source is CNN. He has no real life experience with clinical trial design, is aloof, distant, cocky and divorced. Thankfully, he is still a thorough physician and cares about his patients. His kids are grown and gone.

His neighbor, also an excellent physician is Dr. Bullock (Dr. B), a graduate of Granada's St George's Medical School. Dr. Bullock also has an independent internal medicine practice downtown. He and Dr. Axel play golf together occasionally and this weekend was one of them. Dr. B reads only the *NEJM* and *Annals of Internal Medicine* but takes the time once every two weeks to spend about two to three hours dissecting any journal article on topics he finds interesting. He has even updated his training on how to critically analyze publications through a course he took last summer at an Ivy League school. He is also divorced. His medical news source is to Google search any topic of interest and he does not watch TV.

Both doctors were good friends but on this fateful Saturday morning, they disagreed on the treatment of Covid-19. Dr. Axel insisted that there was no randomized double-blinded, placebo-controlled study showing that HCQ works in Covid-19 infection. Dr. B said that there was sufficient anecdotal evidence in the face of a pandemic to at least try HCQ. Dr. A argued that he wasn't going to ever rely on anecdotal or weak studies to give his patients a drug that has not been proven. Dr. B said true, but no patient is going to sign up to be on the placebo arm of a study, they just want treatment and they don't care about clinical trials. Eventually, they both parted ways, each maintaining his ground. Two weeks later this small city of 6,000 people with only two medical practices, Dr. Axel's and Dr. Bullock's, had their first Covid-19 death. Panic hit. The coroner, another golfing buddy of both doctors, sends them a text late that night alerting them to prepare for the expected rise in Covid-19 cases. Both Dr. Axel and Dr. Bullock's offices were packed full the next day. Luckily they were both ready. Patients stayed in their vehicles for registration and came in based on a number that was posted on a large computer screen at the entrance and visible to most of those in the parking lot. Dr. A's office collected swabs for PCR Covid-19 testing, as did Dr. B's. Patients were reassured and sent back home. The wife, two children and mother of the man that had died of Covid-19 the night before, all came to Dr. A's office with fever and cough for two days. They were also tested, reassured and sent home to self-quarantine and await the test results.

Four days later Dr. B gets a call from Dr. Axel regarding the deceased man's family. They had told Dr. Axel they were switching doctors and would be coming to Dr. B's office. The test results of all four family members had been Covid-19 positive, Dr. Axel added. Dr. B said that's enough reason for them to want to change doctors, you know. "They want me to start them on HCQ and I can't", Dr. A replied. *(Everyone in my house knows I Can't died a long time ago!)* "Why can't you?" Dr. B replied. "It's not been proven, Dr. A responded. What do you lose, Dr. B replied? Nothing, Dr. A responded. What if it works in these patients but you failed to treat them, how would that look in this small town? I haven't figured that out yet. Ok, I'll see them when they get here. Dr. B, caught off guard, quickly performed a Google search and found the Zelenko protocol as well as the pilot study in France done by Dr. Didier Raoult. Later that evening after work hours, Dr. B called Dr. A to inform him of his treatment plan and advised Dr. A to research and read up the available evidence so he could help his patients and forget the media. Rather than follow this advise, Dr. A took offense and blurted out to Dr. B that he went to a better medical school than Dr. B and that Dr. B was in no position to tell him how to read on a disorder or manage patients. Dr. B apologized for making him feel that way but reminded him that his medical school will not tell him what to do at this moment. Only a good friend and colleague would. Dr. B told him to picture what would happen if over the next few weeks, Dr. A failed to treat all the Covid-19 patients that came to his office. All his patients would go somewhere else to get treated with HCQ and whatever is available. Dr. A said that would never happen. Four weeks later, all except two dementia patients, had left Dr. A's clinic. Even Dr. A's nurse, left him. Once it became clear to Dr. A's patients that he had no intention of treating the patients with HCQ and was awaiting randomized double-blinded placebo controlled trials to prove that HCQ works, his patients left. The two patients that stayed would probably have left if they had full cognitive function. In that time 6 more of his patients had died of Covid-19, including a set of healthy 22-year old twins. Dr. Axel decided to report Dr. B to the medical board, by which time his own nurse had left him to start working for Dr. B. She said she left because when she became Covid-19 positive, Dr. A refused to treat her. The economic impact of Covid-19 had hit Dr. Axel before the lockdown was ever instituted.

Someone once said that data is not always evidence and the absence of evidence is not necessarily evidence of absence. If you don't know what to look for, you may not know what you've found.

The basis for using HCQ in Covid-19 alone or in combination with Azithromycin has both anecdotal evidence, evidence from randomized trials, and scientific evidence based on molecular modeling studies that no one ever mentions. The consideration of using HCQ in Covid-19 started with an article titled *Breakthrough: Choloroquine phosphate has shown apparent efficacy in treatment of Covid-19 associated pneumonia in clinical studies report in China (**Gao et al., Bioscience Trends** 2020;14:72-73)*. Shortly after, Dr. Didier Raoult's team published another article titled *Hydroxychloroquine and Azithromycin as a treatment of Covid-19: results of an open label non-randomized clinical trial (**Gautret et al**, 2020 **International J Antimicrob Agents** 2020; 20:105949)*. **In this pilot study,** 42 patients were enrolled of the 48 targeted and 6 were lost to follow up. Primary endpoint was clearance of the virus by PCR. By day 3, 50% of the HCQ-treated patients were negative vs. 6.3% in the control group, and by day 6, 100% of those treated with HCQ and Azi were negative compared with 57.1% of those treated with HCQ alone and 12.5% in the non-treatment control group. Even at this level before all the controversies in the US media began, an obvious gesture on the part of scientists trying to find a way to rescue the world from Covid-19 was taken as a fine gesture. But there is a science behind the findings of this second journal that has been obscured by third parties. Regardless of political leanings or fears of retribution from the media, a few doctors stepped out to share their results in their practices about their success with HCQ or HCQ and Azithromycin but many were booed. Some, like Simone Gold, MD, were fired. But Dr, Fantini et al, did a fantastic job in identifying the molecular interactions between HCQ, azithromycin and the coronavirus. Dr. Fantini and colleagues used molecular dynamics to show that azithromycin and hydroxychloroquine act on specific molecular targets on the virus and host cells to prevent infection. These

81

are undisputable realities showing at the molecular level exactly how azithromycin and HCQ work so that the results of Gautret et al could be predicted with some degree of certainty and why we have 100%, 57.1% and 12.5% primary outcomes in the HCQ/Azi, HCQ and no treatment groups respectively in the Gautret et al study.

The ACE-2 receptor that SARS-CoV-2 attaches to is localized in lipid rafts. SARS-CoV-2 attaches not only to the ACE-2 receptor but also through other domains. The coronavirus depends on certain membrane components such as gangliosides that serve as attachment co-factors to help the virus attach to the host cell. One of these gangliosides is GM1. GM1 is a ganglioside that plays an important role in binding and endocytosis of respiratory viruses and also coronavirus. *(Fantini, Chahinian & Yahi. International J Antimicrob Agents 56 2020. 106020)* There is a ganglioside binding site on the spike protein of the coronavirus found at the tip of its N-terminal domain (NTD). It can attach to the host cell through this ganglioside binding site and not just through the ACE-2 receptor. Both receptor sites therefore present drug developers an opportunity to create molecules that can competitively or irreversibly inhibit virus binding to the host cell. Azithromycin shares molecular similarity with the sugar moiety of GM1 and it can bind competitively by mimicry to this ganglioside binding site on the SARS-CoV-2 virus and prevent infection. What Fantini et al also found was that the N-terminal domain of the spike protein of SARS-CoV-2w has a flat surface for ganglioside binding. According to Fantini et al, when seen from above, the viral spike, consisting of three interdigitating spike proteins to create the corona-like projections seen on electron microscopy. The spike protein has a typical triangular shape with a ganglioside-binding domain at the apex of each triangle and a central area devoted to ACE-2 receptor binding. This means that SARS-CoV-2 binds to the host cell via ganglioside binding sites as well as through the ACE-receptor binding site. This dual binding process has been found in HIV-1 and bacterial neurotoxins. HCQ saturates virus attachment sites on gangliosides in the vicinity of the ACE-2 receptor thereby inhibiting cellular attachment mechanisms. HCQ acts on the ganglioside surface to prevent virus-host membrane interaction while azithromycin occupies the ganglioside-binding domain of the spike protein. The way Fantini describes the SARS-CoV-2-HCQ-Azithromycin complex is that

"if the dimer is compared metaphorically to a butterfly, azithromycin inhibits the QFN triad in the head of the butterfly while HCQ binds to the wings of the butterfly. "

So HCQ and Azithromycin do have a synergistic antiviral effect on SARS-CoV-2. It should be obvious then that both drugs should be given early if they are to be effective and azithromycin can only be given for the 5 to 7 days as seen in some Covid-19 treatment regimens if there is no risk of QT prolongation. Otherwise one or at most two doses of azithromycin should be given at the commencement of treatment with HCQ.

The HCQ Debate, Caxton Opere, MD

18

Skipper et al.,
Annals of Internal Medicine. July 16, 2020
HCQ in Non-hospitalized Adults with Early Covid-19.
Randomized. Placebo controlled
491 patients. Montreal and Minnesota

Randomized double blind, placebo-controlled. Subjects were symptomatic non-hospitalized adults with laboratory confirmation of Covid-19 or probable Covid-19 and high-risk exposure within 4 days of symptom onset. They received HCQ over a 5-day period. Of 423 patients enrolled in the study, 341(81%) had laboratory-confirmed SARS-CoV-2 infection or were epidemiologically linked by exposure to a person with laboratory confirmed infection. According to the journal,

> "of these 341 patients, 145 were PCR-positive for SARS-CoV-2, 280 were known high-risk exposure to a PCR-positive contact; 84 had both. The remaining 82 participants (19%) were enrolled with suspected Covid-19: they had Covid-19-compatible symptoms and reported high-risk exposure, but the contact's PCR was pending or unavailable. Of these 37 had 2 of 3 symptoms of cough, fever, and shortness of breath. Those with a PCR-confirmed diagnosis took a mean of 2.2 days of symptoms to enroll, compared with 1.3 days for those enrolled via symptoms and an epidemiologic link to a PCR-positive contact."

56% were enrolled within 1 day of symptom onset. The primary endpoint of the study was change in overall symptom severity over 14 days. Symptoms and severity were determined at baseline and at days, 3,5,10, and 14 using a 10-point visual analog scale.

This is the HCQ dosing regimen for the Skipper et al 2020 study
800mg + 600mg (6-8 hours later) = 1.4g
600mg daily x 4 days = 2.4g
Total = 3.8g

By the fifth day, 54% (109/203) of the patients in the HCQ arm reported symptoms versus 56% (108/194) in the placebo group. By day 14, 24% (49/201) in the HCQ arm reported symptoms vs. 30% (59/194) in the placebo arm. In the placebo group there were 10 hospitalizations and 1 death, while in the HCQ group there were 4 hospitalizations and 1 death.

According to the authors,

"The HCQ arm had a mean reduction of 2.60 points from baseline on the 10-point visual analogue scale for symptom severity versus a 2.33-point reduction in the placebo group, a difference that was not statistically different. 77% (157/203) of the participants in the HCQ arm reported complete adherence to the regimen versus 86%(166/194) in the placebo group. Based on the study, HCQ did not cause any statistical difference. **16% of participants contributing data to the primary end point had a confirmed negative result on PCR,** and the study may not inform whether an effect would be observed in populations at higher risk for severe Covid-19."

Problem #1: Methodical miscommunication of statistics
The numbers in any statistical analysis can be manipulated to fit whatever you want it to say. So as the authors feel like, they can use statistical analysis to make something that was significant look otherwise. In other words, if an author is biased against a drug, they can always perform a statistical operation that makes any significant positive finding with HCQ look inconsequential, while magnifying any negative association with the drug and you and I would not know the difference. Not only that, the words carved around the statistical analysis can also be manipulated to say something that is not true but which can be readily retracted as if done innocently or without intent. The bold phrase above **"16% of participants contributing data to the primary end point had a confirmed negative result on PCR"** again reveals some degree of questionable integrity. What that statement is saying is basically that 16% of the patients studied and presumed to be Covid-19 positive and probably started on HCQ were actually Covid-19 negative. So what happens when you give HCQ to patients without Covid-19 and you are trying to see if HCQ will cure their symptoms? If their symptoms were secondary to Lyme disease would you expect HCQ to work? Probably not! I chose a tricky one here because a case report of Lyme disease related demyelinating peripheral neuropathy from France *(Lacout et al, Am J Med. 2017)* showed complete resolution of neurological symptoms when HCQ was combined with doxycycline and IVIG (intravenous immunoglobulin) where IVIG had failed before. Isn't that like giving Benadryl to a patient without an allergic reaction or a shot of Rocephin

to a perfectly healthy human being with no need for the drug? What do you call that?

Problem #2: HCQ doses slightly above recommended standard of 2.4g
A total of 3.8g HCQ was given to the patients in this study but look at the incidence of adverse effects. Medication adverse effects occurred in 43%(92/212) patients receiving HCQ vs. 22%(46/211) receiving placebo. With what Dr. Watson would call "only" a 50 percent increase in total dose of HCQ, adverse effects occurred in 43 percent of the patients. Then what do you think is happening to the patients in those studies in which double, triple or quadruple doses of 2.4g HCQ were given to study patients? Do you think the true adverse effect incidence was recorded in those studies? You may decide to go back and look up these studies and see how low the adverse effects they reported were. As a teaser, try to extrapolate if possible, the number of patients that would develop adverse effects in the studies where 5.6g to 18g of HCQ were given.

Problem #3: Is this Study Part of Another Montreal-Minnesota Study by Bouleware
The study treatment appears similar to the Bouleware et al study, which was described as using HCQ in prevention and early treatment in patients already infected without testing a good number of them for Covid-19 before starting HCQ. I suspect there's nothing wrong with splitting up data in this manner so two different articles can be published. The author however failed to mention if the patients and data were split between them in order to publish two different papers. Dr. David R. Bouleware is on Dr. Caleb P. Skipper's paper, this one, and Dr. Skipper is on Dr. Bouleware's paper, discussed earlier in the book. Dr. Skipper's was a study conducted in Canada and the United States and so was Dr. Bouleware's. In both studies, identical doses and dosing regimen were used in both the Bouleware and Skipper studies. Since Skipper et al were measuring symptom severity after HCQ treatment using an analog scale while Bouleware was measuring efficacy of HCQ in post-exposure prophylaxis prevention of SARS-CoV-2 infection. It's possible the same patients were used in both publications. Both studies referenced clinical trials registration with ClinicalTrials.gov number, NCT04308668).

Problem #4: No objective surrogate markers used in the study end points
While subjective markers of symptom improvement are important, in this environment in which the majority of the scientists have been hacked by Cheyenko as seen in previous studies, any study that is using only subjective measures is suspect. There are objective parameters of

disease severity that could have been used to determine whether a patient has improved. For those of us that are clinicians, we occasionally find patients who prefer hospital beddings and food to their own homes. They do not want to go home once they are ready for discharge and objective measures of improvement can often help healthcare providers tell the patients it's time to go.

Problem #5: Visual Analog scale used not validated by any clinical trials

It's easy to manipulate visual analog scales that have not even been verified as to their accuracy in a study like this. It should be getting clear to you by know that most of these studies were intentionally designed to discredit HCQ's utility in Covid-19 infection and they've done a really good job so far.

Problem #6: This was a highly underpowered study.

A study of this caliber and design ought to enroll enough patients so they can be certain of their conclusions. The authors admit they did not enroll enough patients to be confident about their conclusions.

Problem #7: Visual analog scale not a substitute for objective parameters

The visual analog scale is becoming popular among these poorly powered studies. These analog scales have not been validated in any known trials. Age and stage-based approach to randomized clinical trials are necessary and these study lacked both in terms of symptom severity. Hospitalization as an endpoint is inadequate without specific criteria for hospitalization.

Problem #8: Number tested for Covid-19 communicated in misleading manner

Again to see how mentally sleepy authors expect their readers to be, take a look at this statement made by one of the editors of the *Annals of Internal Medicine* regarding Dr. Skipper's study:

> "Although 82% of patients had laboratory confirmed Covid-19 or documentation of close contact with a confirmed case, only 58% of study participants themselves received Covid-19 testing."- Neil Schlugger MD. *Annals of Internal Medicine Editorial. July 16, 2020*

The statement by Dr. Neil Schlugger could have been more clearly stated as

"only 58% were actually tested for Covid-19"

If our goal as communicators and educators is to communicate the truth and as scientists to make sure that the truth we communicate does not leave anything out or create confusion or harm, many of those patients that have died during this pandemic would have survived. You might have heard of the University of Southampton's comments that 95% of the lives would not have been lost during this pandemic if leading scientists and their governments told the truth from the very beginning. Leading an editorial statement with

"although 82% of patients had laboratory confirmed"

gives the false impression that 82% were actually tested. That's the way the brain processes information. Subliminal techniques of suggesting govern how we read most articles and most healthcare providers "scanning" through a journal article would probably presume and go with the first number and interpret the statement as 82% were tested. Most of those reading the Annals of Internal Medicine trust its contents and while 82% could be perceived as far from 100%, and the mind will play its own tricks on us. Since most healthcare professionals reading the Annals highly esteem it and its editors, they will presume that if they only tested 58%, the trusted editors will have flagged it as a bad study.

Problem #9: Placebo Used was a Confounder

In Canada, the placebo tablets were lactose and in the US, they were folic acid 400mcg. Could folic acid administration affect RNA translation and a process of viral replication? Lactose may cause stomach upset in lactose intolerant subjects and thereby simulate the actual treatment side effect in those receiving this placebo in Canada. I don't see why folate was used in the United States because folic acid is important in RNA and DNA synthesis and may affect viral replication. If you think about the use of Remdesivir, a drug initially used unsuccessfully in Ebola, you should be thinking about the scientific reasoning behind the use of folic acid as a placebo. Folic acid may enhance entry of some viruses into the cells. Folate receptor-α is a significant cofactor for cellular entry for the lethal Ebola viruses. (*Chan SY et al, Cell July 13. 2001. Vol 106, issue 1, p117-126*). That means giving folic acid as a placebo to a patient with Covid-19 infection is not a neutral move by the scientists designing this study. Acosta-Elias and Espinoso-Tanguma estimated that pregnant women were ten times less likely to be hospitalized for Covid-19 compared with pregnant women and attribute this difference to folic acid intake. *(Acosta-Elias & Espinosa-Tanguma. Frontiers in Pharmacology, Experimental Pharmacology and Drug Discovery. July 16, 2020).* The authors also suggest that the severity of the Covid-19 infections in pregnant women may be inversely proportional to the concentration of folate in the body. Again, as far back as in 1957, a study by the NIH showed that mice maintained on diets deficient in folic acid were protected from infection with lymphocytic choriomeningitis. *(Haas et al. Virology. Volume 3, issue 1, February 1957. P 15-21).* Folic acid is therefore a confounder and should not have been used in the study as a placebo.

More problems from article reviewers:

Problem #10: Patients that did not start treatment were not excluded from analysis

Even though intention to treat analysis was used, patients that never took the treatment should not been included in the analysis. In supplemental table 2 where the authors compared symptom severity according to medication adherence there were two groups, those that took> 75%(15-19) of the pills and those that took <75% of the pills (1-14). Now, you cannot place the patients that took zero pills and add them to the patients that took 1-14 pills and perform your analysis of adherence and intention to treat using the 22 patients that never started treatment in the HCQ arm or the 13 patients that never started treatment in the placebo arm. Patients were already rightfully categorized as taking 1-14 pills but the calculations were then done using 0-14 pills taken, a completely misleading, perhaps subtle and may be even intentional. You must remove them. However, the moment you do, the HCQ effect becomes magnified significantly. I'm not saying the authors are manipulating data to make HCQ look ineffective but it's beginning to look like that and it is so skillfully done that it took the brilliance of Professors Claudia Paiva Professor Daniel Tausk to sift through this maze of mathematical insanity.

Problem #11: Statistically significant Outcomes Downplayed by authors.

Again Professors Paiva and Tausk state that after rightfully excluding then patients that never started treatment produced a clear 19.5% effect of HCQ over placebo does exist

The HCQ Debate, Caxton Opere, MD

Problem #12: Authors Misinterpreted their own results.
The authors jumped to the wrong conclusion about the lack of efficacy of HCQ for all the above reasons and they admit their study was not strong enough to make the statements it concluded about HCQ's lack of efficacy.

Problem #13: Wrong calculations on Intention to Treat Analysis
No bias exists in excluding patients that never started treatment in both HCQ and placebo arms but including patients that never started treatment in the full analysis will mask the positive effects of HCQ. Both professors equally condemned the methodically concealed positive effect of a drug like HCQ during a pandemic as harmful.

The misinterpretation of this study, whether deliberate or not, is an international disaster. Patients that could have benefitted perhaps even survived without requiring hospitalization ended up hospitalized, perhaps barely recovering full function after the illness and some even died unnecessarily from treatable Covid-19.

19

Million M, et al.
Early treatment of Covid-19 with HCQ and Azithromycin: A Retrospective Analysis of 1061 Cases in Marseille, France
Travel Medicine & Infectious Disease.
Volume 35, May-June 2020

This study came from the group led by Dr. Didier Raoult, the French scientist that first hinted the world about the potential efficacy of HCQ in Covid-19 pilot study involving 26 patients. Dr. Million with Professor Didier Raoult and colleagues reported retrospectively on 1061 confirmed SARS-CoV-2 positive patients treated for a minimum of three days with the following regimen:

HCQ
200mg tid x 10 days
= *6g HCQ total Dose
Azithromycin
500mg day, 1 then 250mg day 2-5

*this study dose is the only one where the investigators gave more than 2.4g total HCQ and still had good outcomes.

Outcomes measured were death, clinical worsening (transfer to ICU or more than 10 days of hospitalization) and persistent viral shedding for more than 10 days. All deaths resulted from respiratory failure.

Since it's all been bad news about HCQ, let's start with the bad news first. Prolonged viral carriage was observed in 47 patients (4.4%) and was associated with a higher viral load at diagnosis (p<0.001). That means the longer you wait before treating, the more virus would have been released, and the longer it might take to clear the virus. Some may still completely clear the virus despite a high viral load on starting treatment. The study reported that a poor clinical outcome was observed in 46 (4.3%) patients, 2.3% of the patients reported a mild adverse effect and 8 (0.75%) died. Virological cure was obtained in 973 patients (91.7%)

within 10 days. Deaths were in patients 74-95 years old thus establishing safety and efficacy parameters for outpatient management of Covid-19 patients. They did not try to be cavalier about people's lives nor act like Nazi scientists trying to conduct placebo studies on sick patients at risk of death from Covid-19. They treated everyone they could as that was the only reasonable thing to do when patients present to a doctor. Is that a crime? Or is it a crime to treat the patients with the only available treatment and then record the findings? No. Nevertheless, Dr. Didier Raoult has been insulted by several journalists and some of these journalists may not even qualify to be medical correspondents for their own magazines. By doing the only reasonable thing an untainted researcher and physician can do, the Gambini vultures have used every possible avenue to attack and try to destroy his reputation. This is a man who has been studying emerging infections for almost forty years. Dr. Raoult is Europe's most cited microbiologist, the seventh most cited microbiologist in the world with more than 2000 publications and 104,000 citations. He was bold enough to insist on treating those who needed treatment rather than sacrifice lives of guinea pigs on the altar of methodology. Thanks to him, the world may never have known that HCQ has any efficacy in early and moderate Covid-19 infections, even if HCQ was not useful later in the course of the illness.

It's important to point out that Dr. Million's team used a dose 2.5 times higher than the FDA recommended doses and still got excellent results. They did EKG's and checked QT intervals before starting the patients on the combination of HCQ and azithromycin. The others didn't and it is unlikely that any of the other investigators studying the efficacy of HCQ have had as much experience with HCQ than Dr. Raoult's team. Their primary goal was to take care of patients, not data or methodology.

20

Tang W et al.
HCQ in patients with mainly mild to moderate coronavirus disease 2019: open label, randomized controlled trial
BMJ 2020; 369:m1849. May 14, 2020
191 patients, 150 randomized

This was an open label study with 191 patients of which 150 were randomized; 75 to standard of care, 75 to standard of care plus HCQ. And always remember, if it's open label, it's not controlled. The mean duration from onset of symptoms to randomization was 16.6 days. 148 (99%) patients had mild to moderate symptoms while only 2(1%) had severe disease. Patients with mild to moderate disease were treated with HCQ for 14 days and those with severe disease received 21 days on the HCQ arm.

> ### HCQ Dosing in Tang et al.
> There were two groups of hydroxychloroquine dosing in the study; a 2-week dosing for mild to moderate disease, and a 3-week dosing for severe illness.
>
> Day 1-3: 1200mg daily x 3 days plus
> Day 4-14: 800mg daily x 11 days (for mild to moderate disease)
>
> OR
>
> Day 4-21: 800mg daily x 18 days (for severe disease)

The primary endpoint was negative SARS-CoV-2 by 28 days and whether patients with severe Covid-19 had clinical improvement by day 28. A negative SARS-CoV-2 meant two negative assays at least 24 hours apart without a positive result by the end of the study. One patient in the moderate disease HCQ group progressed to severe Covid-19 and no patients died during follow up. The most common adverse effect was diarrhea in 7/80 (9%) patients in the group that did not receive HCQ and 21/70 (30%) in the group that did receive HCQ. The authors concluded that the study does not support the use of HCQ in patients with persistent mild to moderate Covid-19. Note the key word persistent. There were several interesting problems with this study. Disease severity was as follows:

Mild disease: Mild symptoms and no pneumonia on imaging
Moderate Disease: pneumonia + Fever, cough, sputum production, or non specific symptoms
Severe pneumonia: SaO2/SpO2 below 94% on room air or PaO2/FiO2 less than or equal to 300.

Problem #1: The introduction section of the paper revealed a political and cognitive bias.
"Such a presidential endorsement stimulated a rapid increase in demand for HCQ". Wrong! It was the fear of dying from the pandemic not the US President's endorsement that triggered the increase in demand for HCQ. The President was one of the most disliked personalities in the world and so why would the same people rush to get HCQ endorsed by a President they detest?

Problem#2: Underpowered Study
The study did not enroll enough patients and cannot be expected to yield conclusive reliable results. The authors admit that.

Problem #3: Prematurely Terminated Study
The study was terminated prematurely in typical Gambini fashion. There is something to gain when studies like this are terminated. Terminating a study prematurely usually wins the favor of the general public as well as the medical community, particularly when the study is announced in a press release. The public thinks they have done something benevolent by prematurely stopping a dangerous or worthless study and the medical community respects their decision to cut their losses and quickly end the study. If the study terminators have enough money and clout, they could secure enough airtime and share their study termination on several news outlets. If you stop a study prematurely, it gives the medical world and the general population a feeling that you were doing something really conscientious.

Problem #4: The Authors bring up the subject of Retinopathy as Toxicity in acute HCQ use
It's still unclear why the authors would suggest acute hydroxychloroquine-induced retinopathy in the short-term use of HCQ for Covid-19. In all other studies but the author's, rarely does any Covid-19 trial extend beyond 10 days. On average, the short-term therapy for this deadly disease with the best results usually lasts 5 to 7 days. Retinopathy, damage to the eyes, should not be mentioned for short-term use of HCQ. That's because acute toxicity of HCQ is more likely to kill you before it makes you blind. Pratyusha Ganne and Renuka

Srinivasan published a case report of a 56-year old man with lupus who had developed chloroquine-induced retinopathy after 7 years of being treated with 2.6mg/kg chloroquine and a cumulative dose of 332g. *(Ganne P, Srinivasan R. JAMA Ophthalmology. 2015;133(5):603-604).* Most patients on chloroquine or HCQ that develop retinopathy do so after 5-7 years of a daily intake of 6.5mg/kg/day even though one paper described ocular HCQ toxicity after only 1.9 months of HCQ treatment. *(Yam JC, Kwok AK: Ocular Toxicity of Hydroxychloroquine. Hong Kong Med J 2006, 12(4):294-304).* While tamoxifen increases the HCQ levels by up to 5 times the normal levels, the short-term use of HCQ is unlikely to cause any permanent ocular damage. So asides from a Gambini propaganda approach, it's not clear why retinopathy was brought up in the use of HCQ in Covid-19.

Problem #5: Initial overdosing of HCQ
Patients in the study received a total of 3.6 g of HCQ in the first 48 hours of treatment. If anyone were to develop acute HCQ toxicity, the patients in this study surely qualify. The high HCQ dosing in the first 48 hours in this study was matched only by RECOVERY and Borba et al. The patients received a total of 50 percent more HCQ in three days than is recommended over a 5-day period from the FDA's withdrawn EUA.

Problem #6: Extended dosing of HCQ for 3 weeks
It's not clear why the authors chose 2 to 3 weeks of treatment as most studies show a maximum of 10 days. It's not surprising that they were worried about retinopathy.

Problem #7: Total study dose of HCQ highest in the world
Patients with mild to moderate disease received 12.4g in 14 days and those with severe disease received a total of 18g in 21 days. This is 500% to 750% higher than the safe dose of 2.4g.

Problem #8: Late initiation of HCQ treatment
Randomization to treatment was initiated 16.6 days after onset of symptoms. Worth thinking about why we start Oseltamivir within 48 hours of symptoms and why the study authors waited an average of more than 2 weeks from the onset of symptoms before starting treatment. The only explanation is the Gambini factor as I cannot accept that the authors did not understand the mechanism of action of HCQ and why it should be given much earlier if any meaningful results were actually sought for. The longer you wait before initiating treatment, the lesser the treatment effect you'll get and this is exactly what happened in

The HCQ Debate, Caxton Opere, MD

this study. The probability of negative sero-conversion was 85.4% in the HCQ group and 81.3% in the control group. It's highly likely that the difference in sero-conversion between both the HCQ treated and control groups would have been much more higher than the absolute -4.2 percent obtained in the study if the authors did not wait for more than two weeks before initiating HCQ treatment. By waiting an average of 16.6 days, all the benefits to accrue from HCQ use have probably all but expired. Even then, HCQ still managed to squeeze slightly ahead by a pitiful -4.2 percent.

Problem #9: Clinical symptoms of Improvement leave some doubts about intentions

The authors measured clinical improvement by resolution of fever and return of oxygen saturation to more than 94%. Resolution of fever was defined as having an axillary temperature of 36.6° C or below. *Healthwise*, a University of Michigan publication, defined a normal oral temperature as 98.6°F (37°C) and that axillary temperature is usually 0.5°F to 1°F (0.3°C - 0.6°C) lower than oral temperature. If you do the simple subtraction it means axillary temperature is between 97.6°F and 98.1°F or 36.4°C and 36.7°C. So as far as Tang et al are concerned, a temperature of 36.7°C means the patient has not recovered! Ridiculous.

Problem #10: Improvement criteria ignored patients with chronic lung disease or hypoxia

Patients with malignancies, heart, liver and kidney disease were excluded. No mention was however made of patients with chronic obstructive lung disease, active smokers, or those on home oxygen. In a well thought out and executed study, it is impossible to ignore these last three, especially when you consider one of the recovery criteria, an oxygen saturation of greater than 94%. So what if the patient has baseline chronic lung disease, or their baseline oxygen on room air before Covid-19 infection saturation was 93%? What if it was 88% on room air and the patient was already on home oxygen before hospitalization? In this study such patients would not be considered to have recovered when they recover and return to their pre-Covid-19 baseline. No mention was made on how they handled such patients and they were not excluded in the criteria in the body of the article.

Problem #11: Anti-inflammatory Confounder Used in Standard of Care Group

While it's okay to use such confounder drugs to save a life if indeed anti-inflammatory agents would be helpful (RECOVERY confirms they are) to lower the risk of death, these confounders compete with HCQ and therefore diminish its treatment effect. Statistical analysis in these biased confounder studies rarely take into consideration the fact that they are diminishing the treatment effect of HCQ that is related to its anti-inflammatory therapeutic property.

Problem #12: Study Sponsored by Vaccine Manufacturer
Shanghai Pharmaceutical Holdings, whose subsidiary *Shanghai Fosun Pharmaceutical Industrial Development Co. Ltd* is the maker of a Covid-19 vaccine (BNT162b1), donated the HCQ used in the study. Talk about a conflict of interest.

Problem #13: Authors called the trial "an open label controlled" oxymoron study
If it's open label, remember, it's not controlled. It's a study loaded with bias.

Problem #14: Discrepancy between Protocol on Website and Study Paper
According to a correspondence from Professor Ricardo Savaris, a professor of ObGyn, the ChicTr.org inclusion criteria were patients with symptoms for 12 days or less from onset to randomization yet the authors had a meant time from onset to and randomization of 16.6 days (3 to 41 days). How did they get to 41 days if only patients with symptoms within 12 days were included in the study?

Problem #15: The authors admit that their study outcomes could not be conclusive
Successful containment of Covid-19 was blamed for inability to recruit enough patients into the study and the authors also admit that the open label created unbalanced dosage adjustments.

Problem #16: Late treatment in wrong group
Hospitalized patients will always remain the least responsive group to HCQ treatment of Covid-19. In the absence of adjunctive therapy with zinc, little or no response should be expected from hospitalized patients with Covid-19 because of basic knowledge of virology, pharmacology and pathology of SARS-CoV-2.

Problem #17: Any conclusion based on false evidence will always be false.

97

The HCQ Debate, Caxton Opere, MD

Tang et al said there is no convincing evidence from well-designed clinical trials to support the use of CQ or HCQ in treatment of Covid-19 event though there are no such studies in existence to prove what he is saying. What the study authors are implying goes somewhat like this:

"There is no well designed randomized, placebo
controlled double-blinded study to show
that jumping out of a moving plane
in the sky with a parachute prevents injuries or death."

You can say this for as long as you want in order to belittle the parachute (HCQ) or its users, but that doesn't mean you'll find anyone outside of "Tuskegee" willing to design such an unethical study. Unfortunately, this is one of the studies that has provoked people to passively "accept" the lack of efficacy of HCQ.

Problem #18: Severe Covid-19 patients were not in original protocol
The authors claim that they excluded severe Covid-19 in the original protocol but later decided to include patients with severe Covid-19! The title of the paper again is

"Hydroxychloroquine in patients with mainly MILD to MODERATE coronavirus disease 2019: open label randomized controlled trial."

So why exactly were they adding SEVERE Covid-19 patients to a paper that was studying MILD TO MODERATE Covid-19 patients? Is it because by adding severe patients, HCQ will be surely guaranteed to look like a failure? Why would an ethical ethics committee approve a change to include severe Covid-19 disease in a paper titled MILD to MODERATE Covid-19 disease?

Problem #19: Clinical Improvement Parameter Suspect
It's still unclear why clinical improvement in patients with severe Covid-19 was even considered to be one of the primary outcomes in a paper on mild to moderate disease. The only possible explanation is that severe Covid-19 patients were added as a smoke screen and once the smoke screen disappears, so will the HCQ benefits of clinical improvement that accrue to the mild and moderate Covid-19 patients cases. Fortunately for HCQ, only 2 patients with severe disease were enrolled in this mild to moderate study! The authors claim the protocol was approved.

Problem #20: Authors Admit Study Not Designed for the majority of HCQ Prescribers

"Our trial could not assess the antiviral efficacy of hydroxychloroquine at an earlier stage such as within 48 hours of the illness, the golden window for antiviral treatment in influenza."

Tang et al, "waited" an average of 16.6 days before initiating HCQ therapy and were studying Covid-19 patients with PERSISTENT mild to moderate not ACUTE mild to moderate illness. This is a strange classification but we'll have to work with it. Persistence of anything has to do with the continued presence of something despite intervention or expected resolution. There was no mention of any prior intervention to justify the use of persistent, and since Covid-19 is a relatively new disease that we still have more to learn about, no one knows what persistent Covid-19 is. Nevertheless, they presented a paper to the medical community and the world at large that subtly equates mild to moderate disease with early disease. That's because when you say mild or moderate Covid-19 disease, you're often referring to early disease. Their patients were not early disease but persistent disease yet they are making us believe that HCQ was not effective in early mild to moderate disease as opposed to the mild to moderate PERSISTENT disease that they studied. The mere fact that the group they studied had mild persistent disease probably meant this group of patients would have survived and done well overall than the average populace because most patients don't last 28 days. These patients probably have something going on well for them that the authors ought to have studied in greater detail rather than publish articles that mislead the world about the lack of efficacy of HCQ in early Covid-19 infections.

Problem #21: Authors Admit that Their Study was best conducted in outpatient settings

Problem #22: More than 90 patients (60%) received Antivirals before starting the study

The authors argue that since both the HCQ and non-HCQ groups received antivirals before randomization, the effect should cancel out. Really? What if the treatment only diminishes the observable treatment effect of HCQ when the antiviral medications were helpful? It's a good thing for the patient but it does not provide clarity for the study interpretation. I'm in favor of whatever helps the patient, but if that is the case, this is a muddled up experiment aimed at simply discrediting

99

The HCQ Debate, Caxton Opere, MD

HCQ. Now we have to hope that the antivirals had no real treatment benefit. Let me illustrate the negative impact of this treatment effect that the authors are downplaying as canceling each other if given to both groups. It's of note that in this unique group with persistent mild to moderate Covid-19, only one patient (HCQ group) progressed to severe Covid-19 disease and no one died.

Let's assume that any reduction in symptoms with a treatment no matter how mild is scored a 1 while no reduction in symptoms gets a score of 0 and that no matter how much the improvement, the maximum score will be 1. Let's also assume that HCQ produces a reduction in symptoms when given to the group but the non-treated group had no reduction in symptoms. If you now give antivirals to both groups and it results in even a slight reduction in symptoms, you have to score the reduction in the symptoms in the non-HCQ group a 1 in each responding patient. Once you do that you have effectively reduced the observable treatment effect produced by HCQ. Antivirals may not be effective but they may produce some clinical improvement that diminishes the observable treatment effect of HCQ. I hope this makes sense that by giving some patients antivirals, all you have effectively done is reduce the efficacy difference between HCQ and what is wrongly called the non-HCQ or non-treatment group. That's the Tang et al study in a nutshell.

21

Mitja et al
Hydroxychloroquine for Early Treatment of Adults with Mild Covid-19: A Randomized Controlled Trial
Open Label. Non-hospitalized patients
Clin Infect Dis. July 16, 2020
293 patients; 157 control, 136 intervention
Mean age 41.6, 201 women (68.6%)
Mean time from symptoms onset to enrolment 3 days
86.7% (254/293) were healthcare workers
53.2% had chronic health problems

The primary outcome was reduction of viral RNA load in nasopharyngeal swabs at days 3 and 7 after commencing treatment. If practicing physicians are getting outstanding results with the use of HCQ in their patients, then it is a complete waste of time to keep doing open label biased studies showing HCQ lacks efficacy. The results of these non-blinded studies so far don't match the outpatient results doctors are getting in their clinics using HCQ. In effect besides the fact that non-blinded studies are ridiculous at this point in the HCQ debate, non-blinded studies are useless when trying to resolve a controversy. Scientists accusing doctors of using HCQ successfully in their Covid-19 patients claim the doctors are not using placebos or blinding techniques. Yet they themselves are carrying out non-blinded studies to prove their claim that HCQ is ineffective. Does that make any sense? At least the clinic doctors are taking care of sick Covid-19 patients and preventing them from getting worse while scientists are poking fingers at those doctors but are unable to provide one solid clinical trial showing that HCQ truly lacks efficacy. Instead they carry out open label trials and call it controlled studies. Again, I must say that there is no such thing as an open-label controlled study. If it's open label, it's not controlled and to say it is, makes it look like the authors are intentionally misleading the reader or that they don't know what they are doing. When you think about the people dying from not being able to use HCQ and would have benefitted from it, you wonder how long this charade of lack of efficacy of HCQ in Covid-19 will go on. There is significant bias and secondary gain to publish junk against HCQ so Big Pharma can bring their "Golden

The HCQ Debate, Caxton Opere, MD

Calf" into the market for trillions in profit. But besides the vaccine with zero safety profile, they have nothing else for early treatment.

I think what any sensible research institute should do at this point is to pack up their bags and go find out WHY HCQ works, in whom it is most likely to work, and admit that they've been tricked into creating substandard scientific papers full of holes that is a poor reflection of their true intellect, experience and achievements. In the case of the RECOVERY study, those giving such lethal doses should be investigated regardless of their reputation. You might find out they fit certain criteria from the Cheyenko plan and have secondary gains from such a poorly conducted arm of the HCQ that basically killed innocent people.

HCQ Dose in the Mitja et al Study
800mg day 1
400mg daily x 6 days
Total dose 3.2g

Problem # 1: No Placebo and a Terrible Excuse for Not Having a Placebo Arm
The authors try to justify their reasons for not having a placebo arm as due to a rush. Not sure if they were thinking of the implications of their study without a placebo arm, the same thing actively practicing physicians are been accused of; not having a placebo arm that validates the efficacy of their claims of efficacy. It might have been sensible to state they did not want to use a placebo arm for ethical reasons, but not because they were in a rush. The rush is no reason to conduct a study poorly.

Problem #2: Rushing to Conclusion
The authors confidently, fist beating on their chest I'm sure, announced to the world that their limping study without placebo and without any blinding convincingly rules out "any meaningful virological or clinical benefit of HCQ in outpatients with mild Covid-19" and that HCQ initiated within 5 days and a media of 3 days was not effective in reducing viral shedding compared with no viral shedding. Not too surprisingly they have several additional problems.

Problem #3: Study Underpowered
The authors admit that they did not enroll enough patients for them to make the assertion that their treatment with HCQ could not reduce the risk of hospitalization. Nevertheless they concluded that HCQ did not

102

reduce the risk of hospitalization! It's strange that despite the millions of patients around the world with Covid-19, many of these authors could not recruit enough patients to their clinical trial.

Problem #4: Authors seem not to understand the meaning of the word "controlled"

They gave themselves credit for designing a randomized controlled study!

Problem #5: They hacked the results by using a questionnaire in an open label study

Not too surprisingly, they observed no benefit in HCQ.

Problem #6: Completely downplayed any positive outcomes with HCQ use

As long as there is data available for manipulation, statistics will help you say anything you want it to say. HCQ doesn't stand a chance under those circumstances. The difference in hospitalization risk in the HCQ group was 5.9% and in the control group 7.1%; the authors stated this was similar. It's negligible but it's also a 20% difference!

Problem #7: Confusing classification of Mild to Moderate Persistent Covid-19

Symptom classification can help provide greater clarity. In this study however, the authors chose to create an entity, persistent mild to moderate Covid-19, without defining what they mean by "PERSISTENT MILD TO MODERATE COVID-19". Different diseases can be classified as mild to moderate and such classifications abound and are often straightforward. But what are the criteria for persistent Covid-19? The authors used this phrase without defining what they mean, at least not one that is easy to find in their paper. That would be an "F" on a term paper.

HCQ seems to have failed in all these studies while HCQ remains an outstanding success in many outpatient clinical practices. A good scientist would want to know why there is such a discrepancy between both groups. The tainted scientist will be glad HCQ doesn't work while the curious one will want to find out why it is working in the few it is claimed to be working. The tainted scientist will design studies that almost guarantee failure of HCQ, and interpret studies to fit the narrative of lack of efficacy of HCQ. The curious scientist will do what's called a segmentation—placing the HCQ success and failure groups into

The HCQ Debate, Caxton Opere, MD

multiple segments that provide a template for further analysis. For example, a good scientist will accept the possibility that HCQ may actually be effective in some early cases, in specific patient groups, and may try to segment these patients by blood levels of zinc, vitamin D3, vitamin C, and thiamine, or by diet, culture, age, race, initial inoculum, or comorbidities. A tainted scientist would do what's called a sanitation—eliminate all possible traces of HCQ's efficacy, while simultaneously using statistics to deceive readers into making the wrong conclusions that fit the scientist's biased narrative.

What if there is significant clinical improvement but no virological clearance? What if the virological persistence is a false positive RT-PCR?

The doctors in practice using HCQ are not paid anything extra to use the drug, unlike oncologists who get a percentage of the chemotherapy drugs they prescribe. The oncologist buys the drug wholesale, sells it to the cancer patient at retail, and gets a 106% allowable markup on the retail price. You probably didn't know that. Virtually everyone knows that cancer treatment is a billion-dollar industry and oncologists make a fortune from selling chemotherapy. Doctors prescribing HCQ have nothing to gain by doing so. It's a cheap drug and some are going all out to make it look like the worst drug on the planet. Even though you cannot tell a doctor not to use a treatment he or she has found effective in managing their patient, imagine the amount of outcry against HCQ use in Covid-19. It's the trillion dollar chess game that has totally ignored reality and tries very hard to limit HCQ use in Covid-19 to it's in-vitro laboratory origins. You will soon find a bunch of pharmaceutical companies coming together like a brotherhood to make sure they make the trillions of dollars from this pandemic. I'm not in any place to stop them. It's business and businesses should prosper. They cannot however control the practice of medicine by paying corrupt scientists to produce substandard and defective papers to substantiate a false claim that HCQ is ineffective in early Covid-19 infection and then try to strong arm doctors away from using it through all manner of tactics possible.

Dr. Robin Armstrong was taking care of 56 residents at The Resort at Texas City, a nursing home in Galveston County. Afraid he might lose them all to Covid-19, he summoned the courage to treat 39 of them with HCQ after receiving consent from them. It appears from the April 14, 2020 article by Jason Whitley that 36 of the 39 patients with Covid-19 did very well, two went to the hospital for issues unrelated to Covid-19 and one remains uncertain. The three residents later died. The article referred to Dr. Robinson as a Republican activist who was however skeptical about HCQ and thought it wouldn't work, the article reported. However the idea of seeing 15% of the nursing home die was not acceptable. The catch here is that all the scientists fighting against HCQ don't care who lives or dies. They'd rather fold their arms and do nothing and wait for magic to come along. Some of them may even have been paid large or small sums of money to design these trials and you will never know the truth. What's worse is that some of them may actually be taking HCQ prophylactically every week or two weeks in secret while those following their advise are dying in droves from Covid-19.

On May 14, 2020, Nick Powell of *The Houston Chronicle* reported that Rick Bright, a top vaccine expert with the federal government, filed a whistleblower complaint alleging that he was given a lesser role after he pushed back against efforts to promote HCQ as a panacea. Why don't scientists come up with an inexpensive, readily available treatment for Covid-19, even if it means repurposing already established and approved drugs with known safety profiles? It's as if there is a senseless determination to rabidly hunt down anyone who thinks HCQ might work or even has a logical scientific basis for suggesting its use.

Your job as a scientist, if you're not engaged in patient care, is to make the world a better place. It's not your place to attack doctors doing their very best and risking their lives and reputations prescribing a drug that does not make the pharmaceutical industry the expected trillions from Covid-19.

The HCQ Debate, Caxton Opere, MD

22

Geleris et al
Observational Study of Hydroxychloroquine in Hospitalized patients with Covid-19
NEJM May 7, 2020; 382: 2411-2418
1446 patients. 70 intubated or died within 24 hours.
*Sponsor NIH. March 7-April 8, 2020

The study was designed to evaluate the association between HCQ and intubation or death at a large medical center, New York Presbyterian Hospital in New York City. Seventy of the patients died or were intubated within 24 hours of admission in the study and were excluded from the analysis.

The primary endpoint was a composite of intubation or death. 811 patients (58.9%) received HCQ and 564 (41.1%) did not receive HCQ. 85.9% of those receiving HCQ did so within 48 hours after presentation to the emergency room.

Treatment
HCQ
600mg bid day 1
400mg bid day 2-5

Azithromycin
500mg on day 1
250mg daily day 2-5

Problem #1: Wrong Timing of Dose Administration
Anyone familiar with the mechanism of action of HCQ will immediately recognize that giving the drug to seriously ill patients hospitalized for Covid-19 is giving the drug too late in the course of the illness. From that you can immediately draw conclusions that HCQ will not provide any real associations the authors were seeking and that's exactly what they found. No association. HCQ is not a super drug that can be given at any phase of the illness and be expected to produce excellent results. Medical school and clinical practice taught us that much. HCQ works at certain phases of Covid-19 infection summarized best under one word, EARLY. Give it early, or forget it.

Problem #2: Wrong Patients

The drug was given too late to patients too sick to benefit from HCQ therapy. How sick were they? Seventy of them died or were intubated within 24 hours! Of the remaining patients, 166 died without intubation and 180 patients were intubated and of these intubated patients, another 66 also died. The patients were so sick 346 patients, that is, one out of every four of them (25.1%) in the study, had a primary endpoint event of death or intubation. Giving HCQ to the sickest patients and expecting a response should be considered medically unsound practice by now.

Problem #3: Misleading Recommendation

To fit the current overall narrative in the media, the authors, fully aware that they were giving HCQ to their sickest patients still concluded that they do not support the use HCQ outside of randomized clinical trials. The authors have no sound basis for making such a restriction or recommendation, however you see it. HCQ is already in use for other conditions and has had an excellent safety profile for more than six decades. Putting such a restriction or recommendation on HCQ would be acceptable if HCQ was a new drug with no known safety profile. HCQ has however been with us for over six decades and is used daily all around the world for many other conditions like systemic lupus, rheumatoid arthritis, malaria and occasionally porphyria. Their study does not provide any scientific reasoning behind restricting HCQ to clinical trials except to tell us there might be the possible influence of the Gambini factor.

Based on what we already know about the mechanism of action of HCQ and the rapidity of sudden deterioration in Covid-19, the most effective time to start HCQ leaves little time left for symptomatic patients other than to start treatment immediately if there are no contraindications.

Problem #4: Admission of Weakness

Study authors say that their study should not be used to rule out either benefit or harm of HCQ therapy. They've rightfully shown us that HCQ does not affect intubation or death, endpoints that strongly suggest things have gone on too long and it is now too late to give the drug. So it's strange as to why they will still recommend the drug be used only in clinical trials. Why even bother using it in clinical trials? Perhaps they suspect that in the end, they may have to come back to HCQ. They could not clarify based on what we already know about HCQ and Covid-19 how HCQ should be used and in whom it will produce the greatest benefit, and in the out patient setting.

The HCQ Debate, Caxton Opere, MD

23

Ferreira et al. 2020.
Chronic Treatment with Hydroxychloroquine and SARS-CoV-2 Infection.
J. Med Virol. July 2020.
Database of patients on chronic HCQ
26,815 SARS-CoV-2 Cases

In this study, Portuguese data on private and public based medical prescriptions served as a database for identifying patients receiving HCQ chronically for management of rheumatologic disorders such as lupus and rheumatoid arthritis. Of 26,815 SARS-CoV-2 cases, 77 patients (0.29%) were on chronic HCQ therapy. After adjustment for age, sex, and chronic treatment with corticosteroids and/or immunosuppressants, the odds ratio of SARS-Cov-2 infection for patients on chronic HCQ therapy was 0.51 (CI 0.37-0.70). According to the authors, the presence of SLE and RA in Portugal is 0.1% and 0.7% respectively and as the authors made clear, patients with SLE have 3.6 times greater increase in herpes simplex infections while those SLE patient on chronic glucocorticoid therapy have 3.9 times greater risk of severe infection than those on HCQ. The use of Chronic HCQ reduced Covid-19 infection by about 50% even though having a rheumatologic disorder almost quadrupled the risk of Covid-19 infection.

24

A Tale of 10 Covid-19 Spouses

So far, none of the clinical trials shown really have convincing data about the lack of efficacy of HCQ in Covid-19. Most of the investigators in these studies humbly admit their work did not have the strength of scientific conviction behind their conclusions. Yet the US media and government are using the same studies like the Brazilian COALITION or Bouleware et al. study as definitive indicators of the lack of efficacy of HCQ in Covid-19. Jumping to such conclusions is not only unscientific, it reflects lack of integrity, because we know HCQ works, they just want randomized controlled trials. Many journalists don't even know what it means except that they've heard Dr. Fauci say it's the only way to be sure that HCQ is effective. Unfortunately it's not the only way. The authors are saying we're not sure if our research findings support the statement that HCQ is ineffective in Covid-19, but since the overall narrative is to say HCQ is ineffective, we're going to go with that common narrative. That's not science, it's group think. Unfortunately such thinking is backed by Boris Cheyenko's journalists and by Big Pharma. What makes the utility of HCQ more confusing in Covid-19 are the intellectual superstars. They are masters in epidemiology, clinical trials design, statistics and scientific methodology. ZDogg MD calls them armchair epidemiologists. They can run circles around you with the same statistical analyses that would make your head spin and make the average practicing physician look like a kindergarten student in a quantum physics class. They know their stuff so well that they can prove to you mathematically that there is no randomized placebo controlled double-blinded study to show that if you don't pay your mortgage, the bank will foreclose on your property. If you follow their advice, you'll lose your house. With respect to Covid-19, if you don't treat patients in need of HCQ with the drug, they may lose their health or their lives. These intellectual "giants" are the biggest challenge to understanding the realities of Covid-19 treatment or the real world impact of neglecting the use of HCQ. I sure wish these masters of clinical trial design would sit down and try to figure out what it has cost the United States to instill fear into doctors now afraid of prescribing HCQ if all we've heard about HCQ's inefficacy are actually lies. Instead they have their armory loaded, ready to blast at the methodology of any study daring to show efficacy of HCQ. However you do not find them attacking the lethally dosed HCQ

The HCQ Debate, Caxton Opere, MD

studies with the same fervor or rage that they do the ones in favor of HCQ, even though the same standard applied to both will show the latter has just as much merit in its conclusion of efficacy as the former anti-CQ studies are portraying a lack of efficacy. Since they are so good at what they do, they forget to include the reality of the clinical significance of the pro-HCQ studies in their raging ripping comments on anyone in favor of HCQ. You'll find them on the internet if you look hard enough, and you'll instantly be able to pick up their arrogance and the likelihood that besides their expertise in methodology, they are really hung up on what they know, not the reality of what is called clinical significance. Let me explain the clinical significance with the story of *The Ten Covid-19 Spouses*.

The Story of Ten Covid-19 Positive Spouses

Imagine ten of your patients in your private practice with Covid-19 symptoms between the ages of 27 and 37 going to the emergency room at the early stages of Covid-19 infection. They do not have any EKG abnormalities and all ten had varying degrees of well-controlled hypertension on one antihypertensive medication. All ten were started on HCQ/ZINC combo rather than the HCQ/Azithromycin, after they were confirmed Covid-19 positive. The emergency doctor said he did that because he wasn't sure if the patients would follow up with their primary care physician (GP) for a recheck of their EKG. Two days later, nine of the ten patients were called by your office staff to find out how they were doing and made appointments for them to come in the next day. They were all feeling better, their fever cough and shortness of breath had resolved but the tenth patient had travelled on a business trip and could not be seen in the clinic that day. He later called to say he was fine. Repeat testing Covid-19 of all ten patients two days later came back negative. Four days later, their spouses showed up in your office with fever, cough and shortness of breath. All ten spouses tested positive for Covid-19 by RT-PCR and they all had fulltime jobs. While they were waiting in their cars, you heard Dr. Anthony Fauci announce on NBC that HCQ is ineffective in Covid-19? Should you believe him and should that stop you from prescribing HCQ/Zn or HCQ/Azi to these ten new patients with Covid-19 whose spouses just got cured with your treatment regimen?

The ten spouses all told you that they would rather take the HCQ/Zinc or HCQ/X combination than do nothing and end up dead, regardless of whatever Dr. Fauci said on TV. A researcher bent on methodology will be paralyzed but a doctor has to treat his patients. That's what clinicians are good at doing better than anyone else, skillfully treating patients.

Scientists do not have to deal with intimate clinical issues patients and their families bring to the clinic. We do. You started five of the ten spouses on HCQ/Zinc and the other five on HCQ/Azi after explaining to them the rationale behind each treatment and what you hopefully expect. This is called "TREATMENT" and is different from "TRIALS". All ten patients had virological clearance in 5 days and complete resolution of fever, cough and shortness of breath in 3 days. So if a doctor treats twenty of his patients in this manner, what exactly has he or she done wrong? Absolutely nothing! If I use a drug in my clinic with excellent results in 100 patients and a well-designed clinical trial with 300 patients shows no treatment or minimal treatment benefit with the same drug, should I just abandon the use of the drug in my patients or should I continue to treat them and continue to expect good results? As far as treating my patients early in the course of Covid-19 infection with HCQ/Azi or HCQ/Zinc, there is a science that backs my treatment and patient outcomes that further substantiate my decision. I run a clinic not a research center. If I have done no harm and the patients improved, as a doctor, I have done what my patients expect of me and what I expect of myself, especially when no one is offering a cure or treatment and the other option is to watch patients deteriorate and perhaps even die. If you want to criticize my approach, first come up with a better option than the one I have given my patients. Passing insults on me for continuing to treat my patients and continuing to get excellent outcomes when nothing else is available means whoever is passing the insults doesn't understand medicine and may be a paid stooge by the Gambini goons. Most of those launching attacks on doctors themselves do not treat patients every day and are probably not in contact with Covid-19 patients regularly. They simply read journals without dissecting the methodologies and if they do treat patients, then they have probably let so many of their patients get hospitalized or die unnecessarily. It's worse when journalists add their insults on doctors to the charade because they do not understand the molecular and pharmacological aspects of Covid-19 treatment strategies. What if the clinical trial has flaws and the investigators themselves are admitting that their clinical trial results are weak and inconclusive? Should I still abandon the drug or drug combination that is effective in my own patients even when I see clear clinical outcomes and an excellent treatment effect? No I shouldn't, except the government through some corrupt agency officials paid by Big Pharma, strong arms me into letting patients die by not allowing me to prescribe the only known effective early treatment for Covid-19. My treatment may not meet the standards of an RCT, but should I abandon my effective treatment because of someone else's research findings? Wouldn't I then

The HCQ Debate, Caxton Opere, MD

be guilty of ecological fallacy if I am trying to apply the results from a population studied to individual cases in an outpatient setting? What if some government officials already paid by Big Pharma want HCQ used only in clinical trials so that they can use statistical methods of manipulating data to diminish the treatment effect? Will you say that is absolutely impossible? We know they can't do that if a doctor in the clinic simply treats his patients with a drug combination and retests them days or weeks later for Covid-19 and reports his or her findings. They can't deny those types of results. But if you do the same in a clinical trial, they'll find fault with something in your methodology that will then be blasted through the airwaves to say your results were invalidated. Just ask Professor Didier Raoult, Yale Professor Harvey Risch or Dr. Michael Zervos of Henry Ford Hospital System in Detroit. Such an overwhelming proof of HCQ's efficacy "must be stopped or suppressed by every means," it seems! It's tiring just listening to the rant from those so far away from treating Covid-19 patients complain about the use of HCQ. They're not exposed to Covid-19 patients and can sit back in an armchair and dictate what others should do.

ECOLOGICAL FALLACY

I used the phrase earlier without defining it. What is ecological fallacy? It's a fallacy in which the results obtained from studying a group is wrongfully applied to individuals. Ironically, when you want doctors treating patients successfully with HCQ alone or in combination with other drugs to accept the results of clinical trials showing a lack of efficacy, aren't you forcing them to commit ecological fallacy? Hard to swallow when your own methods are used on you? You are forcing doctors to practice ecological fallacy.

In the United States, so many people have died unnecessarily because doctors are afraid of prescribing HCQ to patients. Yet the doctors as well as citizens and residents of this great nation keep blaming their President, a man that had already told them to use HCQ for Covid-19. I think Dr. Fauci is responsible for this veil of darkness over the minds of the majority of the doctors in the United States. He has blurted out that HCQ is ineffective and never once admitted that the drug has any efficacy. The Covid-19 infection and death rates in the United States is an embarrassment and a tragedy, yet leading physicians in the United States keep deceiving the masses about the lack of efficacy because they want gold standard, randomized placebo controlled, double-blinded studies to prove the HCQ parachute works. Such folly. Every time I see a patient in the emergency room or the Covid-19 unit about to be intubated, after struggling with COvid-19 symptoms for more than a week before coming because their doctor would not prescribe HCQ, I know the lies of the US healthcare leaders is responsible for that innocent death. Thanks to the overreaching influence of Big Pharma in all aspects of legislation. In fact, this is probably the first time in the history of the United States were a President is independently wealthy he does not have t cater to the needs of Big Pharma and its lobbyists.

No one at this stage is going to be able to design ethically acceptable randomized, placebo-controlled, double blinded studies to prove the efficacy of HCQ or lack thereof. Most of the studies you have seen so far are evidence that somebody is paying another to lower the ethical and scientific standards and present falsified or misleading data to the medical and scientific community as well as the public at large. As a result, many well-meaning doctors are now afraid to prescribe the right drug. While interviewing with Reverend Dr. Winn Henderson for his Covid-19 podcast, he said he had called 35 actively practicing and experienced doctors in North Carolina to find out which of them was prescribing HCQ to their patients. None of these experienced physicians was prescribing HCQ. That just means that based on the Covid-19 infection and death rates, at least 35 patients, one from each doctor, would die unnecessarily, as a result of the doctor's fear of retribution for prescribing HCQ. It's like a prison system. Where is the heart and the caring in them? Journalistic terrorism at its worst has driven doctors into caves of passivity and fear!

Big Pharma Wants Evidence

Anecdotal evidence is never the standard to dictate how medicine is practiced in the modern world. Nevertheless the observation or practices of astute physicians can pave the way for greater discoveries and shed more light on how to better treat what seem like mysterious diseases. Who would have thought that over 90% of peptic ulcers cases was due to an infection with *Helicobacter pylori*. Solid evidence based on randomized, placebo controlled double-blinded trials with proper statistical analysis of predetermined endpoints approved by an institutional review board and decent ethics committee is the gold standard for confirming conclusively that a treatment works. You will not always have that gold standard in order to decide whether or not to treat. As you've seen so far, those who insist on only gold standard studies are unable to produce gold standard clinical trials to show conclusively that HCQ is ineffective in Covid-19. Should we therefore

The HCQ Debate, Caxton Opere, MD

fold our arms and let our patients die of Covid-19 simply because there are no gold standard clinical trials or should we make the most of the silver lining from anecdotal evidence? Which one will save patients from dying or getting seriously ill? Those saying HCQ is ineffective are guilty of double standards and of innocent blood. They are guilty of double standards because they insist that doctors that want to prescribe HCQ for Covid-19 patients provide proof for its use. They on the other hand are using sham studies that do not meet the barest standards to buttress their precariously dangerous position on HCQ's lack of efficacy. They are also guilty of innocent blood because they are forcing busy doctors and other practitioners to doubt the efficacy of HCQ in early use and to shy away from prescribing it to patients that would benefit the most. That is causing many doctors to fold their arms passively watching patients get critically ill and perhaps die from Covid-19. The only thing that makes sense here is that Big Pharma has seen an opportunity to make trillions and will not let their fangs off the meat! To ensure a steady stream of insane profit, Big Pharma pays governments, lobbyists and whoever can be bought. How much do they pay? According to the March 3, 2020 *JAMA Internal Medicine* article *Lobbying Expenditures and Campaign Contributions by the Pharmaceutical and Health Product Industry in the United States from 1999 to 2018* by Dr. Olivier Wouters, $4.7 billion was spent over a twenty-year period. Every year, about $233 million dollars are paid to senators and lawmakers by Big Pharma to ensure they do what Big Pharma wants done. The article breakdown was $414 million in contributions to candidates running for president, congress, national party committees, etc. The paper states that $22 million went to presidential candidates and $214 million to congressional candidates. The article also stated that of the 20 senators and 20 representatives who received the most contributions, 39(97.5%) belonged to committees with jurisdiction over health-related legislative matters. In 2018, according to the article, the US spent about $3.6 trillion dollars, 17.6% of its gross domestic product, on health care, including $345 billion on prescription drugs. Like the saying goes, follow the money! Still wondering why there is a war on the cheap drug that is available all over the world?

The first randomized placebo controlled double-blinded study comparing appendectomy with antibiotics in the management of CT-confirmed acute appendicitis was a Finnish study described in the November 2018 issue of the BMJ. Yet the first successful appendectomy was performed in London on an 11-year old boy on December 6, 1735, almost three hundred years earlier. Why wait that long? The wait was because there was a scientific principle behind performing the procedure. Has anyone felt it was wrong for surgeons who opt to remove an inflamed appendix surgically rather than use antibiotics? No. Even now with the results of randomized controlled trials comparing antibiotics to surgery, the jury is still out *(Salminen et al. JAMA. June 16, 2015)*. When you have a scientific basis for doing what you're doing to help patients using safe effective drugs with an established excellent safety profile, anyone trying to wrestle your arm away from what you're doing, without providing an equivalent or better alternative is suspect. As you've seen so far, most of the "studies" do not meet the standards they accuse clinicians with anecdotal evidence of providing. Most of their arguments against HCQ are presuppositions, egotistic theories with no scientific grounding and statistical analysis often unrelated to the proper care of an actual patient. I never read once on these anti-HCQ websites for the methodology experts how to actually take care of a patient with Covid-19 nor did I detect a hint of compassion in them. Not once did I find a thoughtful indication of what doctors should do with sick Covid-19 patients besides the methodological dialogues and the scorning of those using a drug they have found to be helpful in their patients on these websites. Which brings us to the question of solutions and scientific thinking, a process that can only begin if we ask the right questions instead of arrogance and insults on those using the drug? What if HCQ only works in a specific group? How do we identify that group? What role does HCQ play in Covid-19 treatment when combined with zinc in inhibiting the replication of the virus or is that pseudoscience with no basis?

Joe Brew, data scientist at Hyfe and Carlos Chaccour, Assistant Professor at IS Global co-authored a website article on www.publichealth.team titled *Lying with Data* dated July 30, 2020. In this article, the authors reflected the sentiments of most epidemiologists, misuse of data by those favoring hydroxychloroquine. Their answer after asking the question of whether Ivermectin is useful in Covid-19 therapy is that THEY DON'T KNOW. Imagine telling a patient who needs to be treated for a condition they expect you to manage that YOU DON'T KNOW. Never going to happen. Analysis upon analysis from different websites or epidemiologist blogs regarding the use of HCQ in Covid-19 are consistently clear, if they will admit the truth, that they don't know the answer. I must assume that while they may be so knowledgeable about statistical methods, they regrettably do not treat patients. How then will they ever know? Statistics will not give them an answer, only real patients will.

The HCQ Debate, Caxton Opere, MD

Doctor means you can take the only available information to make decisions that improve the life of your patient (s) no matter how small that data is. Every doctor knows the importance of randomized placebo controlled double blind trials in reassuring the doctor of the treatment he or she is about to administer to a patient. Having such studies takes the guesswork out of your treatment decision. Yet while a data scientist or statistics professor can say they don't know if a drug is useful or not in Covid-19, a practicing physician has to treat patients whether or not there is a cure. Watching and waiting for your Covid-19 patients to die is not a strategy no matter how glorious the science of RCT's is on paper. In the real world, doctors must make decisions to care and treat patients and if statisticians cannot be sure of the efficacy of HCQ while doctors treating patients with it are sure they have an effective drug, who should the patient follow? The statistician who says a drug has no proven efficacy or limited data on efficacy or the doctor who despite seeing the limited data has sufficient scientific grounding and an excellent safety profile to choose to use it off-label?

"Medical Doctor" is not just an arrogant title that you throw in people's face to show your intellectual superiority, but a title that shows you not only have the knowledge but the heart to care for others. PhD's who do not have to care for patients share the same title and so it is possible that some doctors care about patients more than other doctors. Some doctors don't care about patients at all because that's not what their doctor title is meant for.

PROTECT: This is another randomized study with HCQ versus observational support for prevention or early-phase treatment of Covid-19. It is again an open label study. *(Trials 21 Article number: 689 2020).* You can pretty much figure how this clinical trial is going to end.

25

More Studies About HCQ...

While the gold rush scientists are still waiting on gold standards for HCQ and denouncing retrospective or case studies on HCQ use in outpatients, patients in these studies continue to get well. In Covid-19 one reason retrospective studies are valuable is because the patients and doctors taking care of them may not even realize the data they create will be retrospectively evaluated at some point or so soon. The doctors just did some thinking, came up with a treatment plan based on currently available data and went to work caring for patients. Many did not know their work would be mined or analyzed statistically for useful data just months down the road. Weeks or months after they had stopped taking care of the patients, the curtains were pulled back to see how effective their efforts were in treating Covid-19 patients. It's really an exciting time in the history of medicine. Anyone denouncing such results or attacking the treating doctors or blaming them for not following "gold standards" of randomized, placebo controlled double blinded "studies" truly needs a psychiatric evaluation.

In this chapter I am going to provide results from real patients on the use of hydroxychloroquine. The gold standard seekers are more like concrete thinking psychiatric patients with no flexibility. Some of the evidence from retrospective studies, some prospective, some blinded, placebo controlled. These are not projected computerized models or distorted statistics but real data from real patients.

In going forward, you must dredge for the truth about HCQ as it may be covered in a lot of media misinformation. A key tool you will need is the ability to quickly recognize propaganda media and avoid them like the plague. Unfortunately, most doctors had passively caved in to these propaganda news sources long before the Covid-19 pandemic, making it difficult to extricate themselves from misleading information on the so-called false evidence-based medicine about Covid-19.

How To Tell if a Covid-19 Journalist, Reporter or Physician Writer is Corrupted (Gambini)
A few simple questions can help you determine if a journalist is corrupted by Cheyenko and therefore not worthy of your time.

Question #1: Do they share information for and against HCQ or just information against?

If they only share negative information about HCQ, dump them. It's unlikely you'll find one-sided journalists praising the positive attributes of HCQ as there is no one paying for such information to be put out there. When you do, it's probably by someone intending to create some balance from the negative news about HCQ that fills the entire airwaves.

Question #2: Do they insult doctors with a different perspective?

If you see an article written by a journalist, reporter, or writer, insulting or berating a doctor, because that doctor has a different perspective from the ongoing favored narrative on HCQ, dump them. It's unprofessional to insult another human being just because they do not share the common narrative. To insult another doctor who has been trained to examine evidence in a field in which the writer is not trained is not only unprofessional, it belittles the media and the entire journalism profession. If a doctor is treating Covid-19 patients with HCQ and getting results, what qualifies any journalist to pass the insult? A journalist cannot qualify to pass insults on those using HCQ and getting results. It's just plain ignorance and ghetto-like. Pigs fight dirty, and this is just dirty fighting and for what? Getting a few dollars from some Gambini agent? Is the life saved not worth more than whatever the journalist has been paid to lie or deceive the rest of the world? Journalists that do this type of harassing show they have little etiquette and will do anything for money. Today fellow physicians are afraid to treat early Covid-19 patients with HCQ because they're uncomfortable with the use of HCQ since all they know about HCQ is what they hear on the news or see in the PDR. Medicine is a specialty full of deeply knowledgeable human beings entrusted with the lives of the public. We do not endanger our patients even if we give treatments that may sometime seem controversial. In the case of HCQ however, there is no controversy about the efficacy of HCQ, only journalistic terrorism and misinformation sponsored by Big Pharma that has cost many their lives. Just because you're a journalist does not mean you have the right to insult a doctor about an issue on which you have absolutely no depth of knowledge, training or expertise. It raises suspicions about whether or not that journalist works for Gambini. It indicates a complete lack of etiquette and it's clear that doctors using HCQ are going against the grain and not without good reason. A good journalist, like the good scientist, tries to figure out why doctors are doing this and if they have the mind, read the entire articles denouncing the use of HCQ themselves. When something outside of their field is gong on, this will be the first time I will see a journalist insult the expert on a topic that they themselves know little or nothing about, particularly on the use of HCQ in Covid-19. Journalists would often defer to paid or unpaid experts without trying to act as professors of medicine. Unfortunately many of the experts sought for answers on Covid-19 have been tainted and the others untainted are so arrogant and too full of themselves and their theories to lend any practical steps to the HCQ debate. A journalist cannot attack a doctor on medical issues on which even doctors on both sides of the issue cannot fully claim to have all the answers. After all, a journalist cannot simply wake up tomorrow, roll up his or her sleeves and start practicing as a doctor.

Here are some studies, all published in peer-reviewed journals on the true efficacy of HCQ in Covid-19.

1. Effect of Combination therapy of HCQ and Azithromycin on Mortality in Covid-19 **Lauriola et al., Clinical and Translational, doi.10.1111/cts.12860.**
   377 patients studied retrospectively showed a 73% reduction in mortality with HCQ+AZ with adjusted hazard ratio HR 0.27 (0.17-.41)

2. Mortality Risk factors Among Hospitalized Covid-19 Patients in a Major Referral Center in Iran. **Alamdari et al.,Tohoku J Exp. Med, 2020, 252, 73-84, doi:10.1620/tjem.252.73**
   396 patients studied retrospectively in Iran. 93% using HCQ, showing mortality RR 0.45, p = 0.028. HCQ was the only antiviral that showed a significant difference.

3. Use of HCQ in hospitalized Covid-19 patients is associated with reduced mortality. Findings from the observational multicenter **Italian CORIST** study. **Di Castelnuovo et al. European Journal of Internal Medicine, doi:10.1016/ejm.2020.08.019**
   Retrospective study. 3,451 hospitalized patients showed a 30% reduction in mortality with HCQ. HR 0.70 (0.59-0.84)

4. Retrospective study of 307 hospital patients in Ghana. **Ashinyo et al, Pan African Medical Journal, 37:1, doi:10.11604/pamj.supp.2020.37..1.25178.** The study showed a 33% reduction in hospitalization time with HCQ, a 29% reduction with HCQ+AZ, and a 37% reduction with CQ and AZ

5. Implications of myocardial injury in Mexican hospitalized patients with coronavirus disease 2019. **Herberto et al. IJC Heart & Vasculature, doi10.1016/ijcha.2020.100638.**
This is an observational prospective study of 254 hospitalized patients. HCQ +AZ patients had a mortality OR 0.36(p=0.04) and mechanical ventilation OR 0.2 (p=0.008)

6. Clinical portrait of the SARS-CoV-2 epidemic in European cancer patients. **Pinato et al. Cancer Discovery, doi:10.1158/2159-8290.CD-20-0773.**
Retrospective study of 890 cancer patients with Covid-19 had an adjusted mortality HR of 0.41 (p<0.001) in HCQ recipients

7. Covid-19 mortality risk factors in older people in a long term care center.. **Heras et al. Research Square, doi:10.21203/rs-70219/v1.**
Retrospective study of 100 elderly nursing home patients with a median age of 85 years. Mortality in the 70% treated with HCQ+AZ was 11.4% vs 61.9% in the control group. RR 0.18, (p<0.001). All patients had confirmed Covid-19.

8. Early Hydroxychloroquine Administration for Rapid Severe Acute Respiratory Syndrome Coronavirus 2 Eradication. **Hong et al., Infect. Chemother., 2020, doi:10.3947/ic.2020.52.e43.**
90 patients in this study. 42 patients received HCQ 1-4 days from diagnosis and 48 patients received HCQ 5+ days from time of diagnosis. HCQ given 1-4 days from diagnosis was found to be the only protective factor against prolonged viral shedding, OR 0.111 (=0.001)There was 57.1% viral clearance in the 1-4 day HCQ group vs. 22.9% for the 5+ delayed treatment group. Authors state that early administration reduced inflammation d patients should be given HCQ as soon as possible.

9. Outcomes of 3,737 Covid-19 patients treated with HCQ/AZ and other regimens in Marseilles, France. A retrospective analysis. **Lagier et al., Travel Med. Infect. Dis. 101791, Jun 25, 2020.**
This study found that early treatment leads to significantly better clinical outcomes and faster viral load reduction. Matched sample mortality HR 0.41(p=0.048).

10. Markedly Low Rates of Coronavirus Infection and Fatality in Malaria-Endemic Regions – A Clue As to Treatment. **Mitchell et al., SSRN, doi:10.2139/ssrn.3586954.**

The authors looked at developed and less-developed countries and concluded from the impact of Covid-19 amongst 2.4 billion people that those from the more developed and affluent, richer countries were 100 times more likely to be infected and to die from Covid-19. When countries with endemic malaria were compared with those without, the contrast was quite dramatic and showed that those living in malaria prevalent areas were less likely to get infected or die from Covid-19.

11. Efficacy of chloroquine and hydroxychloroquine in the treatment of Covid-19. **Meo et al., Eur. Rev. Med. Pharmacol. Sci. 2020, 24 (8), 4539-4547.**
Authors found that Covid-19 is highly pandemic in countries where malaria is not endemic while Covid-19 is least pandemic where malaria is endemic. An inference that can be drawn from this is the protective effect of anti-malarials. Again, epidemiologists can rip this apart even if it is the only plausible explanation.

12. Covid-19 and Rheumatic autoimmune systemic diseases: a report of a large Italian patients series. **Ferri et al, Clinical Rheumatology. August 27, 2020**
Observational multicenter study of 1641 unselected patient from three Italian geographical areas with different prevalence of Covid-19. A significantly higher prevalence of definite and highly suspected diagnosis of Covid-19 disease or both (OR =4.42; CI 2.93-.65), was found in patients with autoimmune disease particularly those with various connective tissue diseases compared to only inflammatory arthritis (p<0.000) or in patients with ongoing conventional synthetic disease-modifying anti-rheumatic drug treatment.

13. Low-dose hydroxychloroquine therapy and mortality in hospitalized patients with Covid-19: a nationwide observational study of 8075 patients. **Catteau et al., Int J Antimicrobial Agents. Volume 56, Issue 4, October 2020**
Retrospective analysis of Belgian national Covid-19 hospital surveillance data. Patients treated with HCQ monotherapy (HCQ group) were compared with patients treated with supportive care only (no-HCQ group). Death was 804/4542 (17.7%) in the HCQ group and 957/3533 (27.1%) in the no-HCQ group. Compared with supportive care only, low dose HCQ

The HCQ Debate, Caxton Opere, MD

monotherapy of 2400mg was associated with lower mortality in hospitalized patients with Covid-19 diagnosed and treated early (< 5 days) or later (> 5 days).

14. Covid-19 in patients with rheumatic disease in Hubei province, China: a multicenter retrospective observational study. **Zhong et al, Lancet Rheumatology. Volume 2, issue 9, E557-564, September 01, 2020.** The study was done to help understand the susceptibility of patients with autoimmune rheumatic diseases (AIRD) to Covid-19. The overall rate of Covid-19 in the 6228 patients with AIRD was 0.43% (27/6228). The study investigators also identified 42 families in which Covid-19 was diagnosed in either a patient with rheumatic disease or a family member living at the same address between Dec 20, 2019 and March 20,2020. Covid-19 was diagnosed in 63% (27/43) of patients with rheumatic disease and in 34% (28/83) of their family members with no rheumatic disease. (OR 2.68; 95% CI 1.14-6.27), p 0.023, after adjusting for age and sex. Patients with rheumatic disease taking HCQ had a lower risk of Covid-19 infection (OR=0.09; 95% CI =0.01-0.94. p=0.044) than those taking other disease-modifying anti-rheumatic drugs (DMARDs). All patients were taking low-dose to medium dose corticosteroids (5-15mg prednisone equivalent on conversion).

15. Treatment with HCQ, Azithromycin and Combination in Patients Hospitalized with Covid-19. **Arshad et al, Int J Infect. Dis. Vol 97, p396-403, August 1, 2020.** Observational study at the six-hospital Henry Ford Health System in South East Michigan. 2541 patients with a median hospitalization time of 6 days, median age of 64 years, 51% male, 56%African American, were treated with HCQ or Azithromycin or a combination of both drugs. The primary end point was in-hospital mortality and the primary cause of death was respiratory failure in 88%. The overall in hospital mortality was 18.1% (95% CI:16.6-19.7) with the following in-hospital mortality rates: HCQ 13.5% (162/1202), (CI, 11.6%-15.5%); HCQ+Azi 20.1%(157/783), (CI, 17.3%-23%); Azi 22.4% (33/147), (CI, 16%-30.1%): neither drug 26.4% (108/409), (CI, 22.2%-31%)

16. Treating Covid-19 with Chloroquine. Huang et al., Journal of Molecular Cell Biology, Volume 12, Issue 4, April 2020, 322-325,doi.10.1093./jcmb/mjaa014. 22 patients positive by RT-PCR for Covid-19 were treated with either (chloroquine phosphate

(n=10) or Lopinavir/ritonavir (n=12). The CQ group consisted of 3 severe and 7 moderate cases and were treated with CQ 500mg twice daily for 10 days. The Lopinavir/ritonavir group had 5 severe and 7 moderate cases and were treated with Lopinavir/ritonavir 400mg/100mg orally twice daily for 10 days. By day 13, all 10 CQ patients were negative with the first one becoming negative on day 2. In the Lopinavir/ritonavir group, patients started becoming SARS-CoV-2 negative after day 3 and 11 out of 12 turned negative by day 14. The number of patients negative for the virus on days 7 and 10 were higher in the CQ group than the Lopinavir/ritonavir group. The roles were reversed when lung CT imaging was used in evaluating SARS-CoV-2 clearance. Lopinavir/ritonavir resulted in lung clearance imaging of the virus by day 6. By day 9 however, 60% (6/10) of the patients in the CQ reached lung clearance compared with 25% (3/12) in the Lopinavir/ritonavir group. By day 14, all 10 patients (100%) in the CQ group were discharged compared to 6 patients (50%) in the Lopinavir/ritonavir group and patients treated with CQ regained their pulmonary function faster.

In an open letter titled

"Concerns regarding the Misinterpretation of Statistical Hypothesis Testing in Clinical Trials for Covid-19 signed by 38 professor and doctors",

Professor Watanabe and several other doctors complained that the RCT studies for early treatment in outpatients to date show favorable effects with efficacy as high as three times normal when proper statistical analysis was done. Who is responsible for improper analysis of these studies to mislead us because it's time to start asking this question.

123

26

POLITICAL INSANE ATTACKS ON
MEDICAL DOCTOR TRAINING

Doctors think and find solutions to patient's
problems, even when there are none. In
Covid-19, there are none. Let doctors think.

Never has there been such an unintelligent, primitive, ill-directed attack on the practice of medicine as the one we now have in the United States since the onset of Covid-19. Doctors doing their very best to take care of patients while pharmaceutical companies are hopefully trying to figure what can work best against the coronavirus have come under attack. Most people have no idea what makes a doctor special or why they were allotted any special place in society say more than a prostitute. Very few understand what goes on behind the scenes, the secret lives of future medical students, before a doctor emerges from the shadows of residency or fellowship with the title "MD", "MBBS", "MBBCh" and the more recent "OD" or many other titles used for medical doctors. Nature sometimes selects doctors from their early childhood years. Nurture also selects doctors. Everyone that eventually becomes a doctor is driven into the field by something internal and extraordinary. If you observe closely, you'll find that most doctors have a generous combination of all the traits motivational speakers always demand from their audiences. Grit, focus, quickness of mind, sacrifice, reading, memorization, routines, discipline, focus, undeniable perseverance, attention to detail, delayed gratification, and much more. Every doctor has all these traits and much more than these and that's why doctors are respected so much in most societies.

Medical doctors are winners, passionate, intelligent, driven, hard-working, focused individuals and most of us are caring, compassionate and dedicated to helping others in society. Doctors are not only needed in the healthcare industry, they also contribute directly or indirectly to the advancement of any civilization and community. To launch a full fledged frontal attack on the doctors in the United States as has been happening lately because some have chosen to prescribe HCQ raises concerns and is a subtle indicator of a much deeply rooted problem that suggests the foundation of our civilization may be rotted to the core and is now unstable enough to collapse. Doctors sacrificed so much to get to the point where they can start practicing their profession under the strictest rules and regulations of any industry. Yet they do it with love. When journalists with no knowledge or experience about what goes on behind the scenes and the extended training doctors undergo before they can practice start attacking us, society needs to be reminded that becoming a doctor is not easy. We may be humble but we are not gullible. We always know far more than the action steps we take and as doctors, we are capable of holding our own when it comes to making even the most complex decisions regarding life and death surrounded any patient's care. Many can sense the Gambini factor but don't have the luxury of time or money to be fighting the system. I must explain a little bit of what goes on behind the scenes in the making of a doctor so that we're not treated by the media as if we're some common gas pump attendants as some journalists have done in the past several months. I'll give you brief insights at different stages, of the developing mind of a person that eventually becomes a doctor, and how he or she thinks, usually from a very young age, sometimes as early as the age of five.

For the sake of simplicity, I'll divide the aspects of our education and training and eventual experience into five parts A, B, C, D and E. I believe the layperson ought to be aware of the doctor's mindset, training and education as a continuous journey that begins with self-discipline and personal sacrifice from an early age. It's important to understand the mindset of the average medical doctor because it is the mindset required for any nation to move itself from mediocrity to greatness or to recover from any war or the scourges of mother nature. If after this, you still feel doctors ought to be ridiculed and mocked for abiding by the first principles of our calling and profession when prescribing HCQ for Covid-19 patients, that's an indicator of how low we have sunk as a society! We also need to be clear about one major occurrence in the healthcare industry in the United States, that is, doctors no longer control the practice of medicine. They are pawns. That's one more reason why we are where we are today with this pandemic. Perhaps something will be awakened in you to start something that will bring order back to the chaos we have in the healthcare system, but I'm not banking on it. All the steps leading to the title "Medical Doctor" are rigorous, particularly as you go from the elementary steps of wanting to become a doctor (A), to a reasonable mastery of one or more specialties (E).

At step A, a teenager, having decided to attend medical school begins to sharpen their focus, and demonstrate the mental and physical discipline as well as a willingness to learn difficult things. The majority will start showing a full commitment towards the sacred profession of medicine in

125

The HCQ Debate, Caxton Opere, MD

character and conduct. Getting excellent grades becomes the norm not the thing to celebrate. The aspiring medical student takes the difficult subjects and also does very well with difficult mental tasks. Due to the emotional and physical demands of this stage and the absolute focus and discipline required, rarely would you find a drama queen beyond the 9th grade (JSS3, Form 2) that wants to be a doctor. Stage A is the key to whether or not you'll be willing to sacrifice what is required to become a doctor: focus, mental discipline, physical discipline, commitment to learning difficult things, and delaying gratification. What's very interesting about the traits an aspiring doctor commits to at this stage is that few people in life ever reach this level of cognitive awareness and personal commitment their entire life.

The 5 Stages of A Doctor's Mental Development
A: Activated mind
B: Accountable mind
C: Altered mind
D: Agile mind
E: Adaptable mind

At steps B all the way through E, the practicing doctor is created through education, exposure and experience. During these years, the eventual doctor learns about the human body and hopefully the human mind, how the body functions in health and disease, the different structures organs and systems in the body, and how they work in harmony and perfect unity, until a disease process tries to take over. Also learnt during this period are the different disease processes and systems affected as well as the different biochemical processes that can go wrong, any chemicals or drugs that can be helpful in slowing down, reversing, preventing or managing a disease process at its early, intermediate or late stages. Medical school is not just about knowing what drug to use in one condition but to understand disease processes in the body or mind and be able to formulate a treatment plan based on available chemicals, drugs, research, and any other means that constitutes the practice of medicine. For example a hypothyroid patient may be placed on thyroxin while one with an overactive thyroid needs a drug that will block increased thyroid hormone production. Once a doctor understands a disease process, he can choose which agent or chemical he wishes to use in preventing, slowing down, reversing or treating the disease itself. That's what the title "MD" implies, that you now know the human body so well, you can figure out how best to do any of these four things in order to help bring your patient back to normal or near normal as possible and in the shortest possible time, with the least expensive option and the least side effects, preferably by doing no harm

	Who you are	What you Learn	What You Become	Subjects/Courses. Mindset
A	Focus, mental discipline Physical discipline Commitment to learning difficult things	Sciences Humanities +/- Music	Activated mind	Mathematics, Biology Organic chemistry History, English
B	Organize and complete multiple difficult tasks and/or be exceptionally brilliant	Admission to Medical School	Accountable mind	Anatomy, Physiology, Biochemistry, Psychology
C	Certification	Graduation from Med school.	Altered mind	Pathology, Pharmacology, Public Health, Medicine, Surgery, Pediatrics, Psychiatry Obstetrics/Gynecology
D	Doctor of Doctors	Complete Residency Specialty Training Board Certification	Agile mind	Patient care. Learning speed. Integrate clinical knowledge into medical practice
E	Experience	Subspecialty training or Specialty Mastery	Adaptable mind	Ready for any situation Synthesize new treatment strategies. Integrate research knowledge into medical practice. Lead into the future. Skillfully adapt to any situation

whatsoever to the patient. So when the FDA tells a doctor not to use an effective medication and Big Pharma hires witch hunters to attack those prescribing hydroxychloroquine, there is something inherently wrong with the system. These entities expect us to passively abandon the reason why we became doctors in the first place and the inviolable steps that brought us to that point where we now make decisions about how to manage patients and gain their trust. Particularly in the United States where there are highly regulated multiple checks and balances to ensure that a doctor does the right thing, the final arbiter of whether a doctor

The HCQ Debate, Caxton Opere, MD

does the right thing is patient outcomes. This appears to be favorable to those receiving HCQ from their doctor's early in the course of their Covid-19 infection. The NIH has usurped that leading to many unnecessary deaths.

There are several reasons why a doctor in the United States would not just prescribe any drug, particularly if some government officials do not want the drug prescribed. A controversial drug like HCQ, which really shouldn't be controversial, is one that many doctors shy away from even when they know it will help their patients. I'd like to walk you through these safeguards that ensure that at least in the United States, a doctor wouldn't just prescribe anything that doesn't make sense to a patient as the risk of litigation or even criminal negligence is higher in the United States than anywhere else in the world. When pharmaceutical companies want to dictate what we can prescribe as physicians, they have crossed the line and everyone is paying for it with the higher Covid-19 deaths in the United States today.

12 Reasons Why a US Physician Has no Real Incentive to Prescribe Hydroxychloroquine:
1. Doctors get sued a lot in the United States
2. The United States is also a highly litigious society
3. Doctors prescribing HCQ don't get kickbacks like oncologists
4. The FDA doesn't want it prescribed so prescribing it is risky
5. The malpractice risk rises exponentially particularly in an epidemic if the drug HCQ is as dangerous as touted in the medical journals
6. The prescribing doctor's malpractice insurance can rise significantly
7. The patients are likely to complain about a doctor's incompetence to the medical board
8. Use of HCQ in clinic settings or the ER is off-label and not recognized by the FDA
9. No likelihood of 5-star recognition or cruise tickets from pharmaceutical companies
10. The doctor can get fired from the job
11. The doctor can lose his license
12. The doctor will be attacked by media terrorists

In addition, most of the doctors protesting against the restriction of hydroxychloroquine to hospitalized patients are not criminally minded or independently wealthy. They need to work and cannot afford to have their jobs jeopardized or get sued for malpractice. So why would any doctor in the United States despite all the above, still risk almost everything in order to prescribe a drug for patients that are not their relatives or those with nothing to lose suing the doctor? It's only because the drug really works. HCQ, despite all these artificial barriers, works in Covid-19 patients. If the drug doesn't work, patients will be the ones filing complaints to the medical board against the prescribing doctors, not journalists.

When the EUA for HCQ was first released on April 27, 2020, few people were able to detect the major defect in the fact sheet indications for its use. That EUA may singularly have been responsible for the deaths of hundreds of thousands of Americans from Covid-19. The EUA stated that HCQ could only be used in hospitalized patients or those enrolled in clinical trials. The average layperson or even journalist may not understand why any "ordinary" doctor would disagree with the FDA or other people like Dr. Fauci on the use of HCQ but by now you should have seen enough reasons from those clinical trials identified in previous chapters. For that reason, I want to help the non-physicians reading this book understand why a trained physician can disagree with any other recommendations, particularly if they feel their stance benefits their patients. If doing nothing can kill your patient, you must do something. If what you do is helping your patients and it has a clear scientific basis in clinical practice and an obvious measurable clinical outcome, then not doing anything means harming your patient. That's what malpractice is all about. If your patient will die if you do nothing, but you fold your arms and do nothing, knowing deep down on the inside that if you gave HCQ the patient might get better, but for fear of the media and the government, your patient ends on life support and dies from Covid-19, what have you done?

The HCQ Debate, Caxton Opere, MD

27

Tuskegee, Covid-19, and HCQ:
Profit-Based Insanity?

You should not be allowed to get away with an unethical and subsequently misguided phrase such as "controlled" in your research paper if you are reporting an open label study. In a pandemic where patients who do not receive the denounced treatment could have survived but died as a result of not having received treatment because the published article directly inhibits prescribing or administering the drug, the responsible parties for such a publication should be brought to justice.

> *"Open label designs should not be used in phase I trials in volunteers, phase II pilot or pivotal trials or any other trial in which it is ethically, medically and practically possible to use a double-blind design to achieve more reliable data."*

Hydroxychloroquine is not a Maslow's Hammer and most people who recommend or prescribe it for Covid-19 are not doing so because it is the most prescribed drug in their practice but because they are getting results by starting early, exactly where the best scientific minds provide support and proof of HCQ's maximal efficacy.

If all you have is a hammer, then everything looks like a nail. That's the principle behind "Maslow's hammer". Many doctors untrained and therefore not proficient in evaluating clinical studies, thinking it is just too mechanical and rigid a process. Many MD's have therefore opted for the low road and joined the bandwagon of those attempting to display an air of intellectual superiority by discounting the use of HCQ. It is a form of sloth or mental laziness to not be able to critically assess the usefulness of a thing rightfully. It is however unethical if not criminal to be using groupthink as a doctor. That's not how you got to this point in your career.

Every doctor around the world should read Thomas Paine's *Common Sense*, particularly foreign medical graduates in the USA. It will give you an idea of why you should fight this lop-sided attack on HCQ. The puppet masters have methodically crept in, first into our practice, took over the economic advantages and rendered us burnt out 7-on-7-off ragdolls. Half burnt out or fully so, doctors are unable to think critically in sufficient depth to handle a crisis such as Covid-19. We can easily be swayed and for the most part, have been duped.

If doctors don't put a stop to this nonsense about the ineffectiveness of HCQ touted by Dr. Fauci, we will be the first victims as frontline workers. HCQ works. The data has been manipulated to make it seem like HCQ doesn't work. You now know the truth, at least part of it. Physicians and nurses may be at the greatest risk of Covid-19 by virtue of our profession, the first to come in contact with the disease. If we do nothing, we'll be run over by others with less noble agenda. Our families, loved ones, colleagues may all die from Covid-19 or Covid-20! We ought to prevent this from happening.

How many deaths will it take 'til he knows/That too many people have died?
- Bob Dylan

Whenever we choose to ignore the cries and warnings of others because it doesn't affect us proximately in the moment, it will eventually return full force to gravely affect us through the butterfly effect or the law of unintended consequences. When we ignore the cries of doctors taking care of patients who are getting excellent results with inexpensive drugs and we say "give us evidence from randomized double blind placebo controlled trials" as if they or the patients needed for such studies are machines, we will reap the pain of the Gambini machinery in due season. By now, it should be obvious that there is more to the HCQ debate than meets the eye, as if there is a secret war going on. Just think about this for a moment. A doctor discovers that an inexpensive drug may be helpful in a pandemic that is ravaging lives. Rather than figure out why the drug works, who best to give it to, and when to give it, reputable scientists from around the world are summoned to discredit the drug in every possible way. They must have been well paid to be willing to risk their entire reputation on something like this. If a strange drug works, real science does not set out to prove that it doesn't work but tries to explain why it does work, even if it's in just a small segment of the population. Real science doesn't send out an army of scientists to disprove the efficacy of the drug by doing sham studies that are actually guilty of the same methodological flaws they accuse doctors getting results with HCQ of. Real science will try to find an answer to why HCQ works, in who it works best, and the different levels of expected efficacy in different subgroups, not celebrate a lack of efficacy as noted with the RECOVERY scientist comments. Very few scientists are asking why

131

The HCQ Debate, Caxton Opere, MD

HCQ should be working in the first place and that's not scientific. There are so many reasons why a drug may work in one group and not the other, and intelligent science seeks to uncover why, not indict those getting positive outcomes. If you've followed the news over the last several months however, you'll have seen how doctors prescribing HCQ and getting excellent results have been vilified by a tainted media and a bunch of scientists producing weak inconclusive yet media-backed articles. These papers will give you an idea of who has been bought by the Gambini group. That's why you will find a ton of scientific papers denouncing the effectiveness of HCQ and not much elsewhere. One of such articles was the well written May 22, 2020 article on HCQ toxicity published in the Lancet and New England Journal of Medicine that had to be subsequently retracted! On April 22, 2020 on the forbetterscience.com website, Leonid Schneider audaciously insulted Professor Didier Raoult, a dedicated microbiologist with his article:

"Chloroquine Witchdoctor Didier Raoult: barking mad and dangerous. Is the inventor of chloroquine cure for Covid-19, the French microbiologist Didier Raoult sane?"

Leonid called Dr. Raoult a chloroquine witchdoctor and lauded him with a couple of more insults in his article. It's as if Dr. Raoult never graduated medical school the way this journalist ripped him apart and then asked for donations at the end of his paper. The article was scientifically baseless, unprofessional, very emotional, and lacking in civility. Cheyenko was definitely at work in the paper. Thankfully, most of those prescribing HCQ know it isn't a Maslow's hammer. Leonid did get a response from some readers on his web site. The first response was from a "Sirnzee" on April 30, 2020. Sirnzee shared the results of HCQ use in Covid-19 obtained internationally and tried to explain how HCQ worked. It seemed obvious Leonid had an axe to grind, Sirnzee added, and that Leonid could not separate fact from fiction and focus on the real issue that drove the HCQ debate. No one bothered to ponder on what Dr. Raoult's motive was for recommending HCQ but it certainly wasn't money. Something needed to be done quickly to stop this pandemic and expecting gold standard clinical trials proving HCQ's efficacy at those early stages of the deadly pandemic didn't make sense. Even now, who wants to be on the placebo arm of a promising Covid-19 treatment? No one. Was Leonid hired by Dr. Frank Gambini, as he completely ignored the results other doctors are obtaining everywhere else around the world while name calling? We may never know.

In another online article timed to 12:40am EDT, Alex Ledsom, Senior

Travel contributor (not a medical correspondent) on Forbes.com on July 19, 2020, wrote a piece on Dr. Raoult titled:

"Hydroxychloroquine: Europe Turns Away from Doctor Who Championed Drug With "Irresponsible" Study

Irresponsible study? Europe turns away? So treating your patients without a placebo arm because you'd rather save lives with a promising treatment rather than win accolades for using human guinea pigs in a placebo arm during a pandemic is irresponsible? Alex then sites the retracted May 22, 2020 Lancet journal article by Dr. Mehra et al mentioned above, a study so full of holes it is laughable but nevertheless dangerous in its implications and had to be withdrawn. Alex equally cited the RECOVERY study and the Boulware et al study, both of which you've seen earlier in my descriptions of them as full of holes. If Alex were able to properly evaluate those same studies he quoted, one retracted, two shown in this book to be shams, he probably wouldn't have said what he said. Is Dr. Frank Gambini at work here again? As the saying goes, making real world decisions based on some statistics or p values is not proof that Dr. Raoult was wrong.

The attacks on Dr. Raoult and the counterattacks from his defenders, many of whom have never met him, shows there is a war going on against and for the truth. While some are actually treating actual patients suffering from Covid-19 and are concerned they themselves might infect their families, others are propagating non-factual sensational negative narratives about the dangers of the only effective early treatment. What else do we have for early treatment of Covid-19 patients besides the recently identified Bangladesh study of Ivermectin plus Doxycycline combination which was recently shown to have 100% recovery in 5.93 days and negative PCR in 8.93 days compared to HCQ/Azithromycin which had a 96.3% recovery in 6.99 days and a negative PCR in 9.33 days.

Some have speculated that there is a hidden agenda behind all this debate and that they don't understand why there is so much attack on those prescribing or presenting HCQ as a sensible option until we have a definite solution to SARS-CoV-2 infection. It appears as if HCQ is standing in the way of something that has been planned. On May 27, Devon Cole's CNN update at 3:43pm mentioned that the WHO had temporarily halted its Hydroxychloroquine SOLIDARITY trial, based on a sham study published in the May 22, 2020 issue of *Lancet* the same

133

study that was subsequently withdrawn along with its New England Journal of Medicine article on the same topic. This observational study was full of holes. Dr. Anthony Fauci, head of the National Institute of Allergy and Infectious Disease and White House corona advisor probably based his assertions on HCQ's lack of efficacy for the coronavirus on studies like the shamefully withdrawn Lancet article. I have never heard Dr. Fauci mention that HCQ could even be a possible contender for treatment in early Covid-19, perhaps because I don't watch the news. Maybe he had mentioned it in the past. When Dr. Fauci finally made the announcement on July 29, 2020 in an MSNBC interview that was replayed two days later

> "...on trials that are valid, that were randomized and controlled in the proper way, all of those trials show consistently that HCQ is not effective in treatment of coronavirus disease or Covid-19."

It was a nail in the coffin for HCQ. Or so it seemed. Dr. Anthony Fauci's National Institute of Health had sponsored a study in 2005 that was published in Virology Journal (*Vincent M et al, Virol J 2005. Aug 22; 2:69*), showing that chloroquine, a more toxic relative of HCQ requiring, was a potent inhibitor of SARS-CoV-1 infection. What is puzzling is Dr. Fauci's absolute lack of enthusiasm in suggesting, even if it ends up failing, the drug HCQ to the public rather than have the President announce it. The lack of fervor to announce the use of the drug in trials and all the subsequent denunciations and even fabrications of toxicity of HCQ is equally puzzling. Most of the defective studies you saw in previous sections of this book are what Dr. Fauci is calling "the scientific data", studies almost bordering on fraudulence, several of which were using criminally toxic doses totaling in some instances 18g of hydrxoychloroquine. Recall that the FDA had an emergency use authorization with a decent science-based dosing of 800-400x4 regimen and a total dose of 2.4g HCQ. Contrast this dose, with the doses from the "valid scientific" studies Dr. Fauci would have gladly referenced and you'll see that guinea pigs were sent to those trials to be killed or given criminally high doses of HCQ to guarantee it will fail. If there was any real oversight from an ethics committee or institutional review board with eyes wide open, such studies should never have been approved, except of course there is a Gambini factor. If there's any complicity in this manner, I pray it is fully exposed. Just in case you think intended victims will be well protected by the scientific background and training of those on the institutional review board, you better think twice.

Take a look at some of the total doses of HCQ and recognize that the 5-day total HCQ dose of 2.4g is a really good dose approved by the FDA.

When a Professor of Pharmacoepidemiology at the London School of Tropical Medicine and Hygiene can praise a study with such a dangerous HCQ dosing, you know the Gambini team has probably visited him.

Study*	HCQ Total study dose	Multiples of FDA Safe dose (2.4g)	Ref/Comments
ORCHID	2.4g	100%	
Borba MGS et al,	2.7g	113%	Low dose in same study
Boulware et al,	3.8g	158%	
Skipper et al,	3.8g	158%	No harm
Brazilian Coalition Covid-19	5.6g	233%	
SOLIDARITY	8.8g	367%	
RECOVERY	9.6g	400%	
Borba MGS et al,	12g	500%	
Tang W et al,	12.4g	517%	
Tang W et al,	18g	750%	

*Ibid. All the studies have been referenced and discussed earlier in the book.

Contrast the dosages and invariably unfavorable outcomes with that from NYU's Dr. Philip Carlucci's total HCQ study dose of 2g and the vilified Dr. Zelenko's protocol of 2g and you can see a clear contrast and perhaps why the tabled studies above could not see a benefit with HCQ. HCQ will be ineffective with such toxic doses, and if we physicians are not watchful, we will become victims. I'm surprised no one has protested these toxic doses that were designed to ensure HCQ as a potential candidate fails in well-designed trials. You're probably wondering how many patients that could have survived Covid-19 eventually died from direct HCQ toxicity in these studies. So am I. These human guinea pigs in some of these studies were probably acutely poisoned by hydroxychloroquine and may have died horrible besides lonely deaths. Reminds me so much of the Tuskegee experiments. The only difference is that this time the perpetrators are not seeking to oppress and dominate Blacks, but to oppress and dominate Blacks and Whites and initiate global oppression using the healthcare system. This time, it's not just Blacks that are experimental animals, it's everyone, you included on someone's power petri dish. All the doctors that are touting these inhuman studies as the credible scientific data have really been sucked into a black hole of deception that's going to entrap and enslave them and the entire world if care is not taken and the brakes pulled on this fast moving train. The world needs more doctors not just to stand up for what is right, but to share information, understand the right way to

135

The HCQ Debate, Caxton Opere, MD

expose these crimes on humanity.

There is no properly conducted randomized placebo controlled double-blinded clinical trial proving that HCQ is ineffective in Covid-19, none!

Those that were done and given a semblance of having the gold standard of clinical trial design gave toxic doses of HCQ to guarantee it fails as a potential treatment option. Dr. Frank Gambini and his gang are behind it and you should not let them get away for their crimes against humanity once identified. This is not the first time such a crime has been perpetuated on the American people, but this is probably the largest scale. In 1929, Macon County in Alabama, a syphilis survey spearheaded by Dr. Taliaferro Clark who was then head of the Venereal division of the US Public Health Service (USPHS) determined that the incidence of syphilis was about 36 percent. So in 1932, Taliaferro Clark thought it would be a good idea to save the public health service some money by not treating Blacks infected with syphilis. The question we should be asking today is who is Covid-19's Taliaferro Clark?

The US Public Health Service (USPHS) announced that there would be a day of free medical examinations and that many would be treated for bad blood. But treatment for syphilis was withheld. While these poor Black patients presumed they were getting treated for syphilis, they were donating their blood for various tests but had standard treatment withheld from them. At that time the standard treatment for syphilis was to administer arsenic compounds arsphenamine and neoarsphenamine. Sounds familiar? No treatment beyond aspirin and sub-therapeutic doses of mercury were given to the Black patients. O.C Wenger, took over from Taliaferro Clark and was quoted as saying the USPHS has no further interest in the patients until they died. They were more interested in what they would find at autopsy. The plot was thickened by requesting that the Black patients get autopsies and spinal taps done at Tuskegee Institute, to simulate a sense of trust with this Black institution. The plot hatched, Eugene Dibble, MD, Director of the Tuskegee Institute, was contacted by the USPHS, knowing the Black patients would trust a fellow Black doctor. They were just waiting for patients to die. Meanwhile to sweeten the deal and make the deception more ironclad, Eugene Dibble was appointed to work with the USPHS. The authenticity it brought gave Blacks an assurance that they were therefore in good hands with Dibble, a fellow Black man. A nurse, Eunice Rivers was hired from another hospital, John A. Andrew Hospital, to assist as a research assistant. She would also drive the patients to the university for appointments were the patients thought they were getting treated for syphilis but were receiving only aspirin, vitamins and iron. Her job was to also keep an eye on the patients unbeknown to the latter, to ensure they were present at autopsy. Afraid that these Black patients might decide to die at home and never get the autopsy, the USPHS offered free burials and additional funding from Milbank Fund that agreed to pay the fifty-dollar funeral fee, split between the funeral home and the performer of the autopsy. Between 1932 and 1972, the monitored men were closely monitored and too well. Two years into the study, the USPHS went to the nearby Black doctors and requested that they not treat the Black patients in the syphilis study. The Black doctors all agreed. Those were horrible times for Blacks and I'm almost certain any Black doctor that treated could be hung on a tree. When sexually transmitted disease clinics were started years later, the Tuskegee patients tried to get treatment for syphilis. The PHS ran these clinics and they had the names of the blacks in the study. All the Tuskegee men were flagged on a list and blocked from getting treatment. When penicillin was introduced for the treatment of syphilis in 1943, 30 of the original 400 men were able to find a way around the PHS tightened regulatory noose and successfully got treated. My brother in-law married the daughter of one of those thirty men. Many others died. In 1958, 25 years after the study was started, the surviving participants were given $25 dollars and a certificate of appreciation. When Henry Ford Hospital's Dr. Irwin Schatz read about the Tuskegee Syphilis Study in a medical journal, *Archives of Internal Medicine*, in 1965, he wrote back to the editors about the wickedness of allowing or conducting such a study. No one responded.

"Science without conscience is the soul's perdition"
- *Francois Rabelais, Pantagruel*

The father of modern surgical gynecology and past president of the American Medical Association J Marion Sims (1813-1883) performed several gynecological surgery procedures on female slaves without anesthesia. He performed the first successful cholecystectomy, the Sim's repair for vesicovaginal fistulas, and the first artificial insemination to result in a pregnancy. Sim's statute was erected in Bryant Park in 1894 and was the first of its kind for any US physician. Dr. Sims perpetuated the idea that Blacks are impervious to pain.

"...it was cheaper to use niggers than cats, because they were everywhere and cheap experimental animals."
- Harry Bailey, MD, Tulane University

137

The HCQ Debate, Caxton Opere, MD

28

Who Wins The HCQ Debate: The People or Big Pharma?

It is quite obvious from the preceding chapters that there is an unknown factor in the well orchestrated "failures" of HCQ in sham clinical trials that have been labeled "scientific data" and its rejection and vilification. As the saying goes, follow the money. In the first scenario at the beginning of this book, you saw how the CEO of a multinational pharmaceutical corporation planned and began to craftily execute his plan to assure himself of a trillion dollar windfall. What was missing in the plan was the power of the human spirit and the tenacity of those who know how to get the truth out to others, thanks to the power of the internet. Many of the clinical trial atrocities that you've perhaps heard of or read about would not have been possible without the Internet. When Dr. Stella Immanuel rattled the cockatrice's nest, they attacked her headlong and as far as we know, Dr. Simone Gold who had put the group together was fired from her ER job. A journalist writing about Dr. Simone, knowing fully well she graduated from Chicago Medical School and Stanford University Law wrote "she said she is a doctor", as if she would call herself an MD without being one. That's how low the Gambini method will stoop to slime-ball anyone that stands in their way. They've also forgotten another factor, the God factor. Until God says it's okay to reveal your evil plan so people can see who's been hiding behind the mask, evil plots will always fail. If there's any real sinister plot behind everything connected to this pandemic by a group that have so much power and influence, they've just made themselves Goliaths. You know fully well how that story always ends.

When you examine all the evidence and what I'm about to show you in the next few paragraphs, there'll be no doubt left in your mind about the invisible Goliath and their Gambini method. So far there have been frontal and flank assaults on HCQ and its prescribers using press releases, dangerous drug dosing, reputable journals, reputable intellectual giants, government agencies, freelancers, non-governmental organizations (NGO's) and the likes to vilify the drug including lockdowns and misleading announcements on mask use. The EUA given by the FDA to limit use of hydroxychloroquine to late cases is a perfect illustration of the far-reaching influence of the Gambini method.

In an open letter signed by Adnah Munkarah MD and Steven Kalkanis, MD, Executive VP and Chief Clinical Officer and Senior VP and Chief

Academic Officer respectively, of the Henry Ford Health System, they state clearly:

> "*Unfortunately, the political climate that has persisted has made any objective discussion about this drug impossible, and we are deeply saddened by this turn of events. ... To that end, we have made the heartfelt decision to have no further comment about this outside the medical community.*"

This was a letter they painfully had to write, because after publishing an excellently designed and executed study on hospitalized Covid-19 patients, ravenous wolves descended on the Henry Ford System and the authors of the Covid-19 study that included world renowned cardiologist Dr. William O'Neill along with Dr. Samia Arshad, Dr. Paul Kilgore and last but not least Dr. Marcus Zervos. People with no pedigree, property, purity or conscience, often referred to as sons of Belial, are the ones sent to destroy or defame anyone that stands in the way of Dr. Gambini. These wolves descended on Democrat State Rep Karen Whitsett for thanking the US President for suggesting the use of the drug. She had to file a lawsuit against Michigan Governor Whitmer and the 13th Congressional District Democratic Party for trying to deprive her of her right to free speech in thanking the President. Can you imagine that! They've succeeded so far, but Karma has a payday for everyone. A day will come when the world will know who has been working for Dr. Frank Gambini and Boris Cheyenko and, who these two men are working for. Then justice will arise.

God bears with the wicked, but not forever
- Miguel de Cervantes

29

Favorable and Unfavorable Statistics

In the earlier chapters devoted to explaining the clinical trials, you saw how statistics was manipulated like Enron's accountants to say what was not necessarily accurate about HCQ. As the following example illustrates, it is very easy for any statistician to make data in a study say whatever they want it to say, whether positive or negative. This has been done several times in different studies. All you have to do if you don't like a drug is to reverse a difference of 5.1 and 7.9

> ### The 4S Scandinavian Simvastatin Survival Study
> This was a landmark randomized double-blinded placebo controlled study designed in the early 1990's to evaluate the effects of lowering cholesterol in 4,444 patients with high cholesterol (213-309mg/dl) and coronary artery disease. One group would get 20mg of simvastatin and the other group a placebo. A total of 438 people died, 256 (11.5%) in the placebo group and 182 (8.2%) in the simvastatin group. The difference in overall death between both groups was 3.3%, meaning simvastatin reduced the risk of overall death by 3.3%. In the placebo group, 189 (8.5%) died of coronary heart disease (CHD) while 111 (5%) died of CHD in the simvastatin group. Simvastatin therefore reduced the risk of death by only 3.5%. When the drug company published its findings they said simvastatin reduced CHD deaths by 41% and this was perfectly legal as 5% deaths was 41% lower than 8.5%!

To fully appreciate the clinical implications of this statistical malady, I'll share a story of a patient of mine. He was only 55, had a prior 5-vessel coronary artery bypass two years before I saw him, three heart stents at the age of 51, and came in complaining of severe chest pain a week after he had coronary stents placed in his heart. I was quite concerned and after stabilizing him and getting him ready for transfer to the cardiologist, sat down with him and his wife. It turns out he had been terrible with his eating habits, had no real family history of premature coronary artery disease, and a god blood pressure. He had simply presumed that since the cholesterol lowering drug he was taking would reduce his risk of a heart attack by about 40%, that was a good enough number to enable him to keep eating whatever he wanted to eat. I showed him how the numbers worked and that what he thought was a 41% reduction was in reality a 3.5% reduction. He was perplexed. My hope was that he would have a change of heart after that conversation as he hadn't returned to the emergency room for the past 6 months.

You won't find much statistical evidence in favor of HCQ in most clinical trials for the same reason that those performing those studies rely on Big Pharma for grants, connections, scholarships etc. When the preliminary results on Remdesivir vs. placebo were published results were published by *Beigel et al* in the May 22, 2020 issue of the NEJM, I found some things quite interesting. One was the fact that this issue of the NEJM published the retracted May 22, 2020 article on HCQ cardiotoxicity by Professor Mehra. As soon as this Mehra paper was released, WHO cancelled their HCQ study. At the same time and based on the retracted paper, France immediately banned HCQ use in Covid-19. It looked like a perfect setup or may be it was just coincidence. A week later in the midst of protests regarding the quality of the Mehra paper, it was withdrawn. Now standing out alone on the podium was Remdesivir (RDV). Median recovery time with RDV was 11 days compared with 15 days in placebo. Mortality on day 14 was 7.1% for RDV vs. 11.9% for placebo. Looking real good, the investigators now staked their claim on higher ground by stating that the incidence of serious adverse effects was higher, 27% in the placebo group than RDV 21%! What kind of placebo would give serious adverse effects of 27% than the drug. They must be kidding! Even if we believed everything up till that point, how can any rational person believe that a placebo has 1.3 times more serious adverse effects than the actual drug, in this case, Remdesivir.

When everything else fails and the entire Big Pharma realized they have simply held Americans hostage to their ambition to profit in the trillions while costing many their lives and livelihood, they'll have to comeback to basic repurposing using simple drugs and adjuncts like HCQ, Azithromycin, Zinc, Quercetin and vitamins C and D. But it would have been at great cost to human lives. Most countries do not have Big pharma suppressing information and paying out hundreds of millions of dollars annually to congress and lobbying. They will remain ahead on the Covid-19 treatment strategies that are being shut down in the United States.

Not too long ago, ravenous wolves descended on Yale epidemiologist Professor Harvey Risch shortly after his *Newsweek* editorial was published on July 23, 2020 stating HCQ works and should be allowed as treatment for Covid-19. The website www.medpagetoday.com, accused Professor Risch of citing questionable data. The two-dozen colleagues that published an open letter criticizing Professor Risch reminded me of *100 Authors Against Einstein's*. When does a medical correspondent start talking down on a professor of epidemiology on matters that even an average board certified internist would respectfully defer to the Professor? What an amazing world we now live in. We ought to listen carefully and re-examine falsely presented "scientific data" that you now know was published to intentionally mislead but I don't think anyone other than a trained epidemiologist or physician treating patients can see that. If you don't know how far Dr. Frank Gambini will go, just remember Jennings Ryan Staley, MD, the 44-year old Southern California doctor arrested for peddling a combo cure of HCQ, Azithromycin, Vitamin C and Zinc for Covid-19 back in early April 2020. If you understand the science of therapeutics, the only way Dr. Staley would ever have been arrested was if there was someone pulling the strings behind the scenes. Will you arrest a doctor for treating pulmonary hypertension with Viagra because he understood the pathophysiology and pharmacology of the disease and the drug respectively? Dr. Staley figured out exactly how to treat Covid-19 in its early stages and they basically arrested him and destroyed him. Gambini? You bet!

30

Zinc and Why Big Pharma is Scared of HCQ

George Sachs, the CEO of the pharmaceutical company that hired Dr. Frank Gambini and Boris Cheyenko has been having second thoughts after seeing doctor Jennings Ryan Staley get arrested for identifying the cure even without the adulterated clinical trials they were planning to release. George himself has one son and one daughter in medical school. He was feeling uneasy about the witch hunting they had planned when he read the news of the San Diego physician getting arrested. He called Frank but no response, Boris, no response. Apparently both Frank and Boris had figured out that once George saw the news, with his two kids in medical school, he might want to back out of the plan. As far as Boris and Dr. Frank Gambini were concerned, there was no turning back. Soldiers have been recruited, almost a billion has been dedicated to the war chest, lots of profit in it for Gambini and Boris, and therefore the fight must go on.

A Time To Play
Did you ever have a time in elementary school when your class teacher separated two friends so they don't sit together and disrupt the entire class, particularly if these two are always getting into trouble? Well, CQ and zinc are two good friends and if allowed to sit together, are going to make a lot of trouble for the class teacher, Big Pharma, in the school called healthcare industry.

Zinc was studied as a possible adjunct to treating Covid-19 in the NYU Langune clinical trials with positive results. It is recommended for use in Covid-19. The East Virginia Medical School Covid-19 protocol developed by Pulmonary and Critical Care Chief, Paul Marik MD, includes 75-100mg of zinc for prophylaxis, as well as for out patient and inpatient use. But what makes zinc so useful in Covid-19 and how useful is it in any other condition? You'll have an answer to this question shortly and you'll see why it's not just HCQ that bothers the big pharmaceutical companies but the combination of zinc and HCQ together. The use of hydroxychloroquine for some well-known disorders such as lupus, rheumatoid arthritis, and malaria has been well established. But there are some other conditions you may not be aware for which hydroxychlroquine is used and others for which it is being considered as a potential treatment with great promise. Most people are aware that cancer treatment is a multi-billion and perhaps a trillion-dollar business. But did you know that chloroquine alone or in combination with zinc could potentially destroy this cancer industry? Here's why:

In 2009, an article titled was published by Dr. Solomon and Dr. Lee in the *European Journal of Pharmacology*, titled *Chloroquine And its Analogs: A New Promise of an Old Drug for Effective and Safe Cancer Therapies. (Solomon & Lee, 2009)*. In it, they outlined the potential uses of chloroquine as an enhancing agent in cancer therapies. Notice the use of the word therapies and not therapy, the plural not singular, as there is a good reason for this. The authors emphasized the lysosomotrophic property of CQ as an important attribute that could make CQ drastically improve the efficacy of anticancer therapies. A year earlier, the same authors, along with two other authors had published a study showing that CQ-mediated chemosensitization of cell killing effect of Akt inhibitors is cancer specific. They found that an Akt1/Akt 2 inhibitor compound killed cancer cells 10-120 times more effectively when 10μM of CQ was added than when used alone and that CQ is a very effective and cancer-specific chemosensitizer when used in combination with Akt inhibitors. *(Changkun H et al. Bioorg Med Chem. 2008 Sep 1;16 (17):7888-93.)* Then in 2012, Japanese researchers published the results of an in vivo study of using CQ to enhance the inhibition of tumor growth when combined with 5-FU, the standard treatment agent for colorectal cancer. *(Sasaki et al. Anticancer Drugs. 2012 Aug; 23(7):675-82).* That same year, Maycote et al, published an article showing that CQ sensitizes breast cancer cells to chemotherapy independent of CQ's effects on autophagy of the cancer cells. *(Maycote P et al. 2012 Autophagy8: 200-212)* In 2013, it was shown by Zou et al that autophagy, the ability of cancer cells to survive in the face of cellular stress such as during chemotherapy, was inhibited by CQ. CQ increased the expression levels of two proapoptotic proteins, **Bad** and **Bax** and the authors suggested combining CQ with 5-FU for the treatment of colorectal cancer. It turns out that even much earlier in 2010, Dr. Sasaki had published another paper on the benefits of CQ as an inhibitor of autophagy in colon cancer cells and suggested its use in colorectal cancer. *(BMC Cancer. 2010 Jul 15; 10:370)*

What's more, CQ is not just a safe and useful chemotherapy adjunct, it was found to increase sensitivity of cancer cells to radiation therapy. In 2013, Dr. Rojas-Puentes and colleagues treated 73 patients with metastatic brain cancer using radiation therapy in a randomized double-blinded phase II placebo controlled study in Mexico. 39 patients received whole body irradiation (WBI) of 30 Gy in 10 fractions over 2 weeks concomitant with 150mg of CQ for 4 weeks. 34 patients received WBI of 30Gy identical to the first group with a concomitant CQ arm and 55.1% in the control. The only factor that was independently associated with increased overall survival was the presence of <4 brain metastases. No differences in quality of life or toxicity were found between both arms. *(Rojas-Puentes et al, Radiat Oncol. 2013 8:209)* The progression-free survival of brain metastases rates at one year were 83.9% (95%CI: 69.4-98.4) for the CLQ arm and 55.1%(95% CI: 33.6-77.6) for the control arm. Another example of the potential use of CQ is in non-small cell lung cancer treatment. Erlotinib, is an inhibitor of epidermal growth factor receptor (EGFR) tyrosine kinase used in the treatment of non-small cell lung cancer (NSCLC) and several other cancers. Erlotinib is much less effective in NSCLC tumors with wild-type EGFR. Dr. Zou showed that erlotinib induced autophagy, a protective mechanism for cancer cells, in NSCLC cells with wild type EGFR. When CQ was added to wild-type EGFR erlotinib-sensitive and erlotinib-resistant NSCLC cell lines, CQ was able to inhibit the autophagy and thereby enhance the antitumor activity of erlotinib in vitro and in vivo. CQ helped overcome the innate resistance of the wild-type EGFR NSCLC cell lines. Finally, prostate cancer cells resistant to the Akt inhibitor AZD5363 had their tumor killing activity enhanced by adding CQ. *(Lamoureux et al, Clin Cancer Res. 2013 Feb 15;19(4) 833-44).*

It's time to introduce zinc into the picture with CQ. CQ and zinc are good friends and you may have heard or experienced firsthand what the zinc-HCQ combination can do to Covid-19 patients. That's just the tip of the iceberg as far as we know of what is truly possible when the combination is unleashed at the world of diseases. Probably the only ones that don't want to see HCQ and zinc "sitting together" in the same "classroom" are Big Pharma "teachers". Yet the combination of both in their impact will be nothing short of phenomenal. CQ is a zinc ionophore. An ionophore is a chemical that reversibly binds ions in order to transport them across the lipid cell membrane. What's the big deal about an ionophore of zinc and why does zinc need an ionophore? CQ as we have seen has some anticancer activity but a study published in 2014 *(Xue et al. PLoS One. 2014; 9(10):e109180)* showed that when combined with zinc, the combination was cytotoxic to ovarian cancer cell lines A2780. This potential for treatment of ovarian cancer is yet to be fully explored.

The HCQ Debate, Caxton Opere, MD

Let's recap and simplify. CQ has anticancer activity and enhances the antitumor effect of radiation therapy on metastatic brain cancer as well as the effect of chemotherapy on lung, breast, ovarian, colon and prostate cancer. When CQ acts as an ionophore for zinc, it enhances cancer cell death. The cancer industry is a $100 billion industry owned by Big Pharma and threatened by two little friends, HCQ/CQ and zinc. If you were Big Pharma, you would be scared too! That's not all. Imagine the implication of all these potential benefits of CQ in cancer chemotherapy. Zinc has been shown to help treat viral infections and warts, inhibiting their growth both in vitro and in vivo. Here are a few more examples:

B.M Krenn, et al Journal of Virology, January (2009). Volume 83, No.1, p 58-64. Antiviral Activity of the Zinc Ionophores Pyrithione and Hinokitiol against Picornavirus Infections.
Pyrithione (PT) and Hinokitiol (HK) efficiently inhibit human rhinovirus, coxackievirus, and mengovirus multiplication. Early stages of virus infection are unaffected by these compounds. Early stages of virus infection were unaffected by PT and HK but the later cleavage of the cellular eukaryotic translation initiation factor eIF4GI by the rhinoviral 2A protease was abolished in the presence of PT and HK. PT and HK also inhibit picornavirus replication by interfering with proper processing of the viral polyprotein and lead to rapid import of extracellular Zinc into cells as well as the mitochondria. EDTA abolishes the antipicornavirus effects of PT and HK. PT or HK led to a 3-fold increase in intracellular zinc within a few minutes while PDTC elevated intracellular zinc levels six-fold and all three do this via a rapid uptake mechanism. The uptake of zinc into the cells is dose dependent and the presence of more than $2.5\mu M$ PT, $15\mu M$ PDTC, or $62\ \mu M$ HK caused significant zinc uptake after 15 minutes, and these levels are antiviral.

Jing Xue, et al. (2014) Chloroquine is a Zinc Ionophore. PLoS ONE. 9(10): e1091180. Doi:10.1371/journal.pone.0109180.
Chloroquine enhanced zinc uptake by A2780 cells (human ovarian cancer cell lines) in a concentration dependent manner and sensitizes cancer cells to chemotherapy, radiotherapy while also inducing apoptosis (cell death). To determine whether the addition of zinc and chloroquine can kill cancer cells more effectively, A2780 ovarian cancer cells were treated with increasing concentrations of chloroquine in the presence of increased concentration of zinc chloride for 1 hour. Intracellular zinc was barely detectable but increased drastically when chloroquine was added to the culture medium. To ensure that chloroquine does not mobilize zinc ions already present intracellularly and that the increased intracellular zinc is solely due to increased influx

of zinc, the cells were pre-treated with Ca-EDTA, a cell membrane impermeable metal chelator. Once Ca-EDTA was added, intracellular zinc concentrations did not rise. According to this paper, CQ induced accumulation of intracellular zinc ions primarily in the lysozymes.

Aartjan JW et al. 2010. PLoS Pathogens. November 4, 2010 Zinc inhibits Coronavirus and Arteribirus RNA Polymerase Activity in Vitro and Zinc Ionophores Block the Replication of These Viruses in Cell Culture.
Increasing the intracellular concentration of zinc with zinc ionophores like pyrithione (PT) can efficiently impair the replication of a variety of RNA viruses including poliovirus and influenza virus. This study shows that the combination of Zn^{2+} and PT at low concentrations of 2μM Zn^{2+} and 2μM PT inhibits the replication of SARS-CoV-1 and equine arteritis virus (EAV) in cell culture. The RNA synthesis of these viruses is catalyzed by an RNA-dependent RNA polymerase (RdRp). Specifically, Zn^{2+} directly blocked the initiation step of EAV synthesis but in SARS-CoV-1, Zn^{2+} blocked the RdRP elongation. As a confirmation of this mechanism, both actions of Zn^{2+} were blocked when Zn^{2+} was chelated by MgEDTA. In cell culture studies, high Zn^{2+} concentrations and the addition of compounds that stimulate intracellular transportation of Zn^{2+}, the zinc ionophores have been found to inhibit

- **Picorna viruses** – *Lanke K, Krenn BM, Melchers WJG et al 2007. J Gen Virol 8:1206-1217 (PDTC)*
- **Rhinoviruses** – *Gaudernak e, Seipelt J, Triendl A et al 2002. J Virol 76:6004-6015 (PDTC)*
- **Foot and Mouth** – *Polatnick J, Bachrach HL 1978. Antimicrob Agents Chemother 13:731-734. (Zinc)*
- **Coxackie** – *Si X, McManus BM, Zhang J et al. 2005. J Virol 79: 8014-8023 (PDTC)*

Xiangguo Qiu et al. (2016) Prophylactic Efficacy of Quercetin 3-β-O-D-Glucoside against Ebola Virus Infection. Antimicrob Agents Chemother. 2016 Sep; 60(9): 5182-5188.
The flavonoid derivative quercetin 3-β-O-D-glucoside (Q3G) has the ability to protect mice from Ebola infection when given as late as 30 minutes prior to infection by targeting the early steps of viral entry.

Kaushik N, Subramani C, Anang S, et al. (2017). J Virol 2017 November; 91(21) Zinc salts block hepatitis E virus replication by inhibiting the activity of viral RNA-dependent RNA polymerase.

147

This study showed that zinc salts (zinc acetate and zinc sulfate) inhibited the replication of viral RNA in vitro. An increase in the zinc salt concentration further decreased the level of viral sense and antisense mRNA in a dose-dependent manner, with approximately 95% inhibition at 200µM, a concentration way below the cytotoxic levels of 450µM for zinc acetate and 500µM for zinc sulfate. This lower concentration at which zinc salts inhibited viral RNA effectively ruled out zinc-induced cytotoxicity in reducing the level of Hepatitis E viral RNA.

Haraguchi Y, Sakurai H, Hussain S, et al. Antiviral Research. Volume 43 Issue 2, September 1999 p123-133. Zinc acetate, zinc chloride, zinc nitrate, cadmium acetate and mercury chloride, showed anti-HIV-1 activities by inhibiting HIV-1 RNA transcription.

Read SA, Obeid S, Ahlenstiel C, Ahlenstiel G. The Role of Zinc in Antiviral Immunity. Advances in Nutrition, Volume 10, Issue 4, July 2019. Pages 696-710.
Zinc is an essential trace element crucial for growth, development, and maintenance of immune function. It affects hundreds of key enzymes and transcription and its deficiency is quite common in both developing and developed countries. "An abundance of evidence has accumulated over the past 50 years to demonstrate the antiviral activity of zinc against a variety of viruses, and via numerous mechanisms. Zinc deficiency was first discovered by Dr. Prasad et al over 50 years ago in a group of malnourished individuals presenting with hepatosplenomegaly, dwarfism, hypogonadism and an elevated risk of infection. It enables gene transcription and is a catalytic component of approximately 2000 enzymes encompassing all 6 classes- hydrolase, isomerase, ligase, lyase, oxido-reductase, and transferase. Zinc is biologically essential for cellular processes, including growth and development, as well as DNA synthesis and RNA transcription. Although zinc possesses direct antiviral properties as seen in influenza, it is also critical in generating both innate and acquired (humoral) antiviral responses. Intracellular zinc and extracellular zinc are tightly regulated such that Zn 2+ represents a fraction of total cellular zinc (0.0001%). The vast majority of zinc remains bound to zinc-binding proteins such as serum albumin or intracellular metallothionein proteins. Zinc transport is principally mediated by 2 groups of proteins: the ZnT [solute-linked carrier 30 (SLC30A)] family and the ZIP (Zrt- and Irt-like proteins (SLC39A)] family. The ZnT family is responsible for efflux of zinc outside the cell or influx into organelles. The ZIP family performs the opposite role, transporting zinc into the cytoplasm from extracellular sources or cellular organelles. There are more than 30 human proteins responsible for zinc homeostasis ensuring

balance and preventing toxicity but excess zinc can still lead to copper deficiency. Upon taking a zinc supplement, an increase in protein-bound zinc in the bloodstream is internalized by cells in various tissues and organs through the ZIP transporters. Interferons stimulate an influx of zinc into the target cell. The antivirus properties of zinc are viral specific. The effect of zinc on HSV-1 and -2 have been studied for over 40 years suggesting that zinc plays an inhibitory role on almost every aspect of the viral life cycle

> Viral polymerase function
> Protein production and processing
> Free virus inactivation

Zinc was shown to inhibit HIV-1 replication as far back as 1991 (*Zhang ZY et al. 1991. Biochemistry (Mosc). 1991; 30(36):8717-21 Zinc inhibition of renin and the protease from human immunodeficiency virus type 1*) and also to inhibit viral transcription as far back as 1999. (*Haraguchi et al. Antiviral Res. 1999; 43(2): 123-33. Inhibition of HIV-1 infection by zinc group metal compounds*) but has received little attention, perhaps because of the ambitions of those trying to create an AIDS vaccine. Unfortunately, when the AIDSVAx showed 66-78% effectiveness in African Americans exclusively, the vaccine wasn't given much publicity.

Al-Gurairi FT et al. Oral Zinc Sulphate in the treatment of recalcitrant viral warts: randomized placebo controlled clinical trial. Br. J Dermatol. 2002; 146(3): 423-31.
Viral wart clearance improved after 1-2 months of oral ZnSO4 10mg/kg 600mg max per day

Yagboobi et al. Evaluation of oral zinc sulfate effect on recalcitrant multiple viral warts: a randomized placebo-controlled clinical trial. J Am Acad Dermatol. 2009;60(4):706-8

Let's look at a few studies of the effect of zinc supplementation on viral warts. While several studies have shown the effectiveness of topical and oral zinc in the treatment of cutaneous warts, **Lopez-Garcia et al in the British Association of Dermatologist's publication** *Clinical and Experimental Dermatology Volume 34, Issue 8, December 2009*, claims this was too good to be true. This claim feels like the Gambini propaganda drug denunciation strategy. Lopez Garcia's article basically renounces the effectiveness of zinc in the treatment of recalcitrant viral warts. It was under lock and key and I wasn't really interested in

149

subscribing to the journal and find the sponsors or if the paper had any financial conflicts of interest. Yet despite this unfortunate claim, a systematic review of wart treatments for cutaneous warts almost 3 years later in November 2012 by Simonart & de Maertelaer in the *Journal of Dermatology Treatment 2012; 23(1):72-7* showed that providing zinc supplements was the most effective treatment for cutaneous warts. Does it then make sense that Raza et al had also reported a high incidence of zinc deficiency or lower levels of zinc in patients with persistent viral warts? *(J Coll Physicians Surg Pak. 2010;20(2):83-6.* It does! And to add some icing to the cake, two independent studies, one by *Al-Gurairi et al (2002. BMJ)* and the other by *Yagboobi et al (2009 J Am Acad Dermatol)* showed that the greatest responses of viral warts to zinc therapy were in zinc-deficient patients. Perhaps the parallel may be drawn here that the greatest response to the HCQ-Zinc combination for Covid-19 treatment will be amongst zinc deficient patients while positing that hydroxychloroquine alone would be most effective in prophylaxis, for early treatment in and outside the hospital in patients with normal or high levels of zinc. This could be a worthy research concept in the absence of the Gambini factor. But Big Pharma has everyone under a spell r cage.

Kim JH, et al Gynocol Oncol. 2011 Aug;122(2):303-6. A pilot study to investigate the treatment of cervical human papillomavirus infection with zinc-citrate compound (CIZAR®). Of the 194 women diagnosed with high-risk human papilloma virus (HR-HPV) vaginal infection without evidence of high grade squamous intraepithelial lesions by Pap smear and colposcopy, 76 were treated twice weekly with self-administered intra-vaginal 0.5mM zinc citrate solution containing CIZAR® for 12 weeks. The 76 women in the treatment group as well as the 118 women in the control group were then evaluated for clearance of the HR-HPV infection. After 12 weeks of zinc citrate, 49 out of 76 patients (64.5%) had clearance versus 15 of 118 (15.3%) of the 118 untreated control that had spontaneous clearance. (OR 0.079; 95% CI 0.039-0.165 p=0.001).

Zinc does not cross the lipid cell membrane readily and requires some help from ionophores. There are several ionophores, some of which have been used since the Covid-19 pandemic. HCQ is one of the ionophores allowing zinc influx into the cells. Another ionophore is quercetin.

While zinc has been shown to affect viruses, there is a bacteria that zinc affects that attracted my attention, *Streptococcus pyogenes* also known as *group A streptococcus* (GAS). According to an article on *The Global Burden*

150

of group A Streptoccal Diseases published in **Lancet Infect Diseas. 2005 Nov; 5(11):685-94**, the prevalence of severe GAS disease is at least 18.1 million cases, with 1.78 million new cases each year. The article reports 163,000 deaths annually, over 616 million cases of GAS pharyngitis, 111 million cases of pyoderma, making GAS a significant cause of disease and death globally. Zinc is an essential micronutrient for GAS and zinc homeostasis plays a major role in the pathogenesis of GAS infections. Zinc is required for GAS virulence but the host immune system attempts to override the zinc benefit to GAS by using either zinc deprivation or zinc poisoning to overcome GAS infections. To this end, GAS has also developed mechanisms for addressing the two extreme conditions: GAS has a zinc-expelling mechanism when the host defense uses zinc poisoning as a protective strategy, and a zinc-influx mechanism to combat the host immune defense's zinc deprivation approach to eliminating infection. GAS can adapt to the host's zinc deprivation or toxicity attacks by reprogramming its metabolic processes and even engaging transcription strategies at the genetic level. *(Chandrangsu, Rensing, & Helmann. Nat Rev Microbiol. 2017 Jun; 15(6):338-350).* At the molecular level, all of this looks like a chess game between two grandmasters, bacteria and human, and GAS is a versatile organism causing infections in virtually every human body cavity. *(Makthal & Kumaraswami. Metallomics. 2017 Dec 1;9(12):1693-1702).* Zinc is useful in bacterial infections in innate immunity but some smart bacteria work around it. Zinc oxide nanoparticles have also been shown to have strong activity against *Streptococcus pneumonia* at a minimal inhibitory concentration of 40µg/ml by inhibiting the bacterial biofilm.

Besides engaging in the fight against bacteria like GAS or *Streptococcus pneumonia*, zinc is involved in several cellular processes essential for survival and reproduction such as DNA repair and replication, transcription and RNA translation. In coronavirus infection, zinc reveals its versatility in combining its influence at the transcription and translation levels. When zinc enters the SARS-CoV-2 infected human host cell, it prevents the coronavirus from further replication by blocking the action of RNA-dependent-RNA-polymerase (RdRp). RdRp is the enzyme that allows SARS-CoV-2 to use your protein synthesis factory inside your cells to produce more coronavirus particles. How quickly would you want to block that process? As quickly as possible! Zinc blocks this enzyme once it enters the infected cell (as does Remdesivir). Imagine you're a Hollywood or Nollywood movie star with over 10 million followers and have just released a movie that hit blockbuster records on the opening weekend. Now, picture what happens when you

151

look in a mirror, record yourself on camera, play it back, and download it on your social media channel where raving fans have been promised this particular clip. Over 1 million people had said they would watch the video clip if you posted it. You record the video but you can't get the video to download on your YouTube channel. All because you could not find the UPLOAD button! What zinc does to coronavirus is somewhat like preventing the virus from uploading its selfie on its YouTube channel by deleting the "record" button. If you can't record, you can't post the video and you can't get a million views and likes (additional virus particles).

The power of zinc in combating some of our greatest and stubborn health problems, viruses and cancer, is tremendous and I confess that I didn't' know this metal was that powerful until the pandemic hit. When a study treatment shows benefit and there is no other option but that treatment, would you go with the treatment or just fold your arms? If you did that with a Covid-19 patient without knowing which category of the 80-15-5 your patient belongs to, you might be gambling and not providing patient care.

31

Governments, Vaccines and Bradykinins

In the fall of 1999, Dr Wouter Basson, head of South Africa's Chemical and Biological Weapons (CBWP) and a highly respected scientist in Apartheid South Africa, was arrested on charges of genocide and murdering 229 people, all Black. The CBWP's plan was to develop a biological weapon that would kill only blacks. Basson received a lot of assistance from US scientist Larry Ford, MD and other scientists. Dr. Ford travelled several times to South Africa, teaching the security forces how to poison groups of people and contaminate small simple objects like toothbrushes and kitchen utensils with poison. Ford committed suicide on March 2, 2000, by which time his South African accomplice in the killing of hundreds of blacks, Basson, confessed that he received a lot of help from the United States. Dr. Daan Goosen, former director of the military Roodeplat Research Laboratory in South Africa, confessed during the Truth and Reconciliation Commission hearing in summer of 1998, that biological weapons that would kill only blacks was been sought for. Maybe back then, blacks were thought to be the problem, but what if someone wants to see if a biological weapon could kill Blacks and Whites and Covid-19 is simply a test run? Don't think that only totalitarian governments with military dictators like Hitler, the Communist parties or Apartheid regimes can carry out dangerous experiments on its citizens or sanction private institutions to do the same without fear of prosecution. If you do, it's time to rethink. Just listen to the news, and hear how poor countries are doing well with Covid-19 despite limited resources while America is under siege from the pandemic. Heads of institutions using their influence to deride the only treatment available at this moment seems odd. This book addresses facts not conspiracies and so I want to give you a few insights into things you can read up on your own such as the Manhattan Project, MK-NAOMI and MK-ULTRA.

Very much like the 1929 Tuskegee Syphilis Study, the Kennedy Krieger Institute (KKI) in Baltimore conducted a study in 1992 using children of low-income parents as guinea pigs. In this "Repair and Maintenance Study" as elucidated in Harriet Washington's award winning book *Medical Apartheid: The Dark History of Medical Experimentation on Black Americans from Colonial Times to the Present*, the researchers from KKI met with Black families in 108 housing units with peeling lead paint. The goal of the researchers was to make sure these children eat the sweet-tasting but toxic peeling lead paint and then monitor their lead levels and brain development as these children gradually developed toxic lead levels and showed neurological or other systemic damage. Parents of these low-income children were offered $15 without telling them their children will be exposed to toxic peeling lead paint. KKI researchers also promised to pay for the lead abatement of 125 rental units with peeling pain if the landlords would rent to families with little children. Harriet detailed in her book how one-year old Ericka Grimes had a lead level of 9mcg/dl, a normal reading on April 9, 1993. By September 15, 1994 Erick'a lead level was at a toxic level of 32mcg/dl. According to the *AMA Journal of Ethics Virtual Mentor. November 2003, Volume 5, Number 1*, the KKI study "stemmed from the government's desire to find a less costly means of lead paint abatement because the expense of full abatement was too high compared to the worth of the properties". The Institutional Review Board (IRB) that approved the KKI study protocol was Johns Hopkins University! The courts felt that the IRB, rather than protect the human subjects, in this case, innocent little children, tried to assist KKI researchers to get around federal regulations. The court of appeal stated in no uncertain terms that a vulnerable child will not be used to test potentially dangerous theories better left to a subject who is well informed independent adult. So when an independent well-informed group of physicians say they will not take a Covid-19 vaccine, and attempts to enforce unsafe vaccines upon them through legislation are put in place, covertly sponsored by those intending to profit from mass vaccinations, they are trying to get around the same principle of self-determination.

If you're going to prescribe hydroxychloroquine for your patients be sure to apply clinical principles, be aware of side effects, monitor your patient appropriately and follow a regimen that reduces likelihood of toxicity, preferably the one the FDA used and be sure to look up EVMS protocols, Zelenko protocols, and never be afraid to prescribe. Read widely, probably more than you've ever done before and formulate a treatment plan for the early and later stages of Covid-19 that ensure all your patients will get the benefit of your training, experience and knowledge rather than die from Covid-19 or develop long-term complications such as myalgic encephalitis/chronic fatigue syndrome (*Moldofsky & Patcai, 2011*). FDA's removal of the HCQ for use in Covid-19 may be a stark reflection of how deep Dr. Frank Gambini has sunk his claws into the jugular system of the healthcare system of this nation and

I hope he or she gets caught and is brought to justice. At least seventy medical experiments were brutally conducted by the Nazis on humans and seven thousand victims have been reported. The victims were Jews, Poles, Gypsies, political prisoners, Catholic priests and many prisoners of war. Twenty-three scientists that included administrators and doctors were placed on trial. Seven were sentenced to death and executed because their crimes were so heinous, it was not worth leaving them alive. Josef Mengele, also known as the Angel of Death, was a Nazi doctor at Auschwitz concentration camp that escaped to South America. Did you know that shortly after World War II, a study conducted by Dr. Paul Hahn at Vanderbilt University intentionally gave radioactive material to 829 pregnant women and told them they were receiving vitamins that would improve the health of their unborn babies? Seven children subsequently died of cancers with no similar incidence in the control group. So I know that the current President in the White House, no matter how much he is hated, will not allow such experiments on humans to be conducted on his watch. No matter how hard Big Pharma's influence, he would rather fight them than pretend that such atrocities do not exist.

Vaccine Development

It will be unfair in the HCQ debate not to mention at least one or two important things about vaccines and their development. In 2017, after a 7-year litigation the UK court system awarded damages from the swine flu vaccine to 27-year old Aoief Bennett who developed narcolepsy from GlaxoSmithKline's H1N1 swine flu vaccine, Pandemrix. It's presumed that the FDA, CDC, NIH and DHHS have the best interests of the American people at heart and that they would have put their best brains together to figure that an early vaccine is quite possibly a dangerous experiment on the human race. Why do I say that? The science and the data is why! In order to develop a safe vaccine, the vaccine must first be tested in mice, then in pregnant mice. You then follow the offspring of the mice to see if they develop any adverse effects that the parent did not develop during or after pregnacy. How long you follow the mice is subjective and not fixed in stone. If it appears safe in mice, you will then advance to primates, that is, monkeys. You inject male and female monkeys and again follow them. If it appears safe, then you inject the vaccine into pregnant monkeys, female of course! You must then follow the pregnant monkeys for adverse effects and follow the offspring of the

155

The HCQ Debate, Caxton Opere, MD

monkeys for some years. The only time you halt the safety study is if you find dangerous or unacceptable adverse effects such as neurological complications, birth defects or other serious abnormalities. When that happens you simply terminate the vaccine program. However, if you don't see any adverse effects, you can advance the study to healthy adult human volunteers. You vaccinate the adults, observe them for adverse effects and follow them for a good while to be sure that they do not develop serious adverse effects in the organs, psychological problems, or even cancer. When you deem it safe in healthy adults, you can then test it in females in their reproductive years. Again you have to provide sufficient time to study the potential side effects before moving to the last three groups, pregnant women, children, and the elderly. If you inject pregnant women with the vaccine, you must be patient to observe the women and their babies for adverse effects throughout their pregnancy, and for many years following the birth of the child. You must evaluate the developmental milestones of the child while studying the adverse effects. If the vaccine passes successfully through these stages, you have a winner. From this simple description, you can see that it takes real time, a lot of time, to develop a safe vaccine. This is the informal description. The whole point of this is to prove to the FDA that the vaccine is not only effective but that it is also safe in humans. When you hear or read about any experienced or leading scientist saying that a vaccine that is just a few months old is safe, you know you're dealing with a callous and reckless human being, one that doesn't care much about the lives of others. Just look at the number of people that have died from Covid-19 in the United States alone to date. It is over 200,000! Then ask yourself if there was anyone in this country that could have prevented these deaths by providing a different narrative than the one we've been told to believe in the last nine months.

The average duration of a human pregnancy is 280 days, monkeys, 175 days, mice 21 days.

If you add all the three pregnancy numbers up, you get 476 days. Even at the barest minimum, it would be impossible to have a safe Covid-19 vaccine available within 15 months of the first case. Whoever is pushing for the vaccine does not have any love for the human race and is doing so for profit or something more sinister.

Below is a brief description of the formal vaccine development process once it has a proven safety profile in mice and monkeys.

156

PRECLINICAL. Test in tissue culture and cell culture. Then perform animal testing in mice and monkeys. You vaccinate the animal and then challenge with the virus. Many vaccines fail at this point, as the vaccine usually will not protect the vaccinated animal from the infection. If it succeeds, then you proceed to determining safety and immunogenicity. This phase usually takes a minimum of 1-2 years. Once you vaccinate the volunteers without challenging them, you may proceed to applying for an Investigation New Drug (IND) license with the FDA as well as the approval of your study protocols from your institutional review board (IRB) for the clinical trials you intend to carry out. If FDA approves, then you enter the phases below. This is just a sketch and more details are required.

PHASE I. Safety and stability. Efficacy in terms of generating the right immune response. Does the vaccine need stabilizers, adjuvants or preservatives. 20-30 volunteers.

PHASE 11. Randomized. Blinded. Placebo controlled study to determine safety, efficacy, immunogenicity, method of delivery and schedules. About 100 people are studied. At anytime, the FDA may decide that it is in the best interests of the human race that the study be terminated.

PHASE III. Randomized double-blinded placebo controlled study to determine safety in large groups. Determine adverse events and reporting. 1000 – 10,000 or more volunteers. If adverse effects are 1 in 10,000, you will need to enroll 60,000 people, half in the control group. *(Plotkin et al, 2008).* Measures of efficacy would include disease prevention, infection prevention, antibody production and a host of other immune responses. If everything goes well, then, you can apply for a *Biologics License*. This stage takes about 3- to 4 years.

"By the time the product is offered to the public, it has been studied for a least 15 to 20 years (sometimes longer) in tens of thousands of study participants, by thousands of scientists, statisticians, healthcare providers and other personnel, and has cost at lest $1 billion dollars to produce."
- Paul A Offit, MD, Vaccine Education Center, Children's Hospital of Philadelphia. October 21, 2019

PHASE IV
Once your vaccine is on the market, the government demands continuous safety monitoring to detect those long term or rare adverse effects that may not be detectable in smaller numbers of patients or

157

during early administration. The term for this is post-marketing survey. For example, if only 1 in 50,000 will develop a particular complication, and you only tested 35,000 patients in your clinical trials, you may not have enough patients to see that adverse effect. Again if it will take twenty-two years for major adverse effects to occur in 50% of the people who received the vaccine, a 20-year duration may yield no victims. To this end the CDC and FDA have a reporting system called *Vaccine Adverse Event Reporting System* (VAERS) through which healthcare professionals and consumers can report a suspected vaccine adverse event. This is also complimented by the *Vaccine Safety Datalink* (VSD), consisting of about 6 million members in six health maintenance organizations on the West Coast who may have received the vaccine and can be used as controls or subjects in post-marketing surveys for vaccines.

In July 1902, the United States Congress enacted the first modern legislation, *the Biologic Control Act,* to control the quality of vaccines and drugs. Since the inception of the *United States Public Service Act* of 1944, you will need a government license in order to produce a vaccine or biologicals. The goal of such governments was to protect its citizens. With all this, you can see that except someone is deeply interested in testing unsafe vaccines to depopulate the world through vaccine adverse effects, expecting a safe Covid-19 vaccine in 2022 is ludicrous. The only real competition to vaccines is HCQ and the media is methodically destroying HCQ's reputation. I have been curious about this phenomenon for sometime.

Safety of vaccines in humans requires that studies be done in pregnant primates before testing healthy volunteers and then healthy humans and advance to testing children and pregnant women volunteers before recommending the vaccine for the general population. Forcing people to get vaccinated reeks of a more hidden agenda, one likely concocted by the Gambini method. A pregnancy takes 9 months and you must do this study. Get the idea. Antibodies are not necessarily protective and initial phase 1 studies showing rising titers may mean absolutely nothing in the real world of infection and re-infection. There is no proof just yet that the vaccines will trigger protective antibodies. In the vaccine studies done, the antibody titers are rising but that does not mean the antibodies will be protective. As a matter of fact, there is potential for a dangerous phenomenon called antibody dependent enhancement (ADE) of viral infection described in COVID-19: PHYSICIAN TREATMENT STRATEGIES. In ADE, the coronavirus uses the antibodies you have developed from a prior infection or perhaps vaccination to enhance its attachment to receptors on the host cell wall and enter the cell and cause a more severe infection than if you never received the vaccine. or had the infection. These are phenomena that have to be clarified. The question is would you trust scientists giving toxic doses of a drug with an established safety profile in phase 3 clinical trials to do the right thing with a vaccine?

Every true researcher delights in analytical processes that lead to discoveries, not in shutting down through brute force and regulations, the creativity or suggestions of others.

Vaccines take time to develop and we must wait till the exacting studies are done before providing them to people. The idea of rushing a vaccine without gold standard safety measures means this is a gold rush that may damage millions. There are so many therapeutic agents for early and late Covid-19 but the early ones seem to hold the greatest promise. Unfortunately for Big Pharma, these early use drugs do not offer them trillion dollar profits but so what? They'd rather let us die while they harass HCQ users and then try to come up with an expensive drug? Look at Lagos, a highly densely populated city in Nigeria with over 14 million residents in Nigeria. Lagos has an area of 999 square kilometers and a population density of 14000 people per square kilometer. New York City has a population density of 38,242 people per square kilometer. Nigerians were not dying on the streets from Covid-19 as predicted by Melinda Gates despite such a high population density in Lagos and nothing near the deaths in New York City. Yet Lagos does not have the infrastructure of New York and in some houses, up to 30 people may share three or four rooms. What made the difference in Covid-19 infections and deaths? HCQ. Even though some Nigerians overdosed on CQ, many used it judiciously and Covid-19 isolation and quarantine centers where infected individuals were held, gave the drug with very high success rates.

Covid-19, Bradykinins and Cytokine Storms

Bradykinin and Lysylbradykinin are chemicals often called polypeptides that have been shown by computer simulations to be partly responsible for the symptoms seen in Covid-19 patients. Remember that it was computer simulation that was used, not real patients, in case you get too deeply sunk into the theoretical model of the Bradykinin hypothesis.

The HCQ Debate, Caxton Opere, MD

Some actually feel that what has been called a cytokine storm may in fact be a Bradykinin storm instead. I agree that this may well be what is responsible for the "storm". However if this were the only storm, Tocilizumab should not be effective in severe Covid-19 cases, nor should HCQ. If Bradykinin is solely responsible for all the symptoms and signs of Covid-19 illness, HCQ will not be effective in early cases or at all. Nor would Azithromycin. As you can see, HCQ and Azithromycin have been shown to have specific actions in Covid-19 using molecular dynamics and in real patients. There is however nothing to say that the manifestations of Covid-19 cannot be due to both cytokines and bradykinin and probably even other factors. It's however important to keep treating patients and prevent them from dying and not mix our theoretical inclinations with the reality of what our patients needs as the debate on cytokine-bradykinin storm may distract us from the reality of patients dying. Bradykinins behave like histamine and increase vascular permeability, constrict visceral smooth muscle but relax vascular smooth muscle. Kininase II is the enzyme that inactivates bradykinin, a nonapeptide and lysylbradykinin, a decapeptide, by removing Phe-Arg from the carboxy terminal. Kininase II is the Angiotensin Converting Enzyme ACE-2 and its level reaches almost 200 times of normal in Covid-19. The actions of the kinins are more vascular, so the vascular reactions in Covid-19 could be attributed to them. The "blue toes" due to in Covid-19 have been attributed solely to bradykinin but two cytokines, TNF-α and TNF-β are cytokines that can also cause vascular thrombosis that present as blue toes. As you can see, it is time to put our medical brains together and come up with what will help our patients rather than relish in divisive ventures. The thick jello-like material found in the lungs of some Covid-19 patients on autopsy has been thought to be due to high levels of hyaluronic acid in the lungs. Hyaluronic acid absorbs about 1000 times its weight of water and once it is inside the alveoli, you can see how it draws water into the air exchange space, effectively drowning the patient in their own fluids. The proponents of the bradykinin storm have proposed that since interleukin levels found in terminal Covid-19 patients is low, it means that cytokine storms cannot be responsible for the symptoms in the illness. That's however not the only way to think of interleukins in deceased patients. What if the gel-like material in the lungs serves as an adsorption surface for the interleukins? Was the gel like material assayed to see if its content of interleukins is high or lower than elsewhere in the body? What if exhaustion is why interleukins are diminished in the terminal patients? What if a drop in interleukin is really an ominous sign of impending death? The whole idea is that we should think as scientists not as political opponents. Your ideas plus mine produces something far greater, synergistic and more helpful. I think this lack of cohesive energy is why Covid-19 has had such an impact in the US more than elsewhere to date.

Both cytokines and bradykinin may be simultaneously responsible for the Covid-19 pathologies. Why does it have to be one and even though Ockham's razor may push us to consider only one agent, that may still be linear thinking that could set us back by months if we don't' consider all the options and start treatment immediately to save as many lives as possible! We should not however forget that the entire Bradykinin theory came from a government simulation study.

The HCQ Debate, Caxton Opere, MD

32

The Ideal HCQ Clinical Trial

Let's say the grass on your lawn has an abundance of a naturally occurring chemical that prevents or cures diabetes, hypertension, high cholesterol, cancer, heart disease, and asthma. You can cook or chew as much of this grass as you want and no one will bother you. The moment you decide you want to sell this grass to the public however, you will have to go through a regulatory agency for approval as a treatment for these ailments. For example, evaluation of the safety and claims of usefulness (efficacy) for any new medications and medical devices is carried out mandatorily by the Food and Drug Administration (FDA) in the United States, the Medicine and Healthcare products Regulatory Agency (MHRA) in the UK, and their equivalent in other countries such as BfArM in Germany. They scrutinize every claim to a treatment or cure a drug manufacturer makes, to ensure the safety of their citizens. And guess who pays for this evaluations, you! You want to sell your grass, go ahead. Just know that the 4S study cost an estimated $162,206,600 (www.quora.com) before the cholesterol-lowering drug simvastatin (Zocor®) could reach customers. You will have to manufacture the drug(s), recruit patients as well as doctors, researchers, chemists, statisticians, etc. Then you will have to test the drug in animals and then humans. God help you if animal activists get wind of your desire and can locate your lab!

Besides these regulatory agencies, there are usually two major groups involved in any drug clinical trial; those that will give the drug(s) to be tested to others, and those that will receive the drug(s) to be tested. The former group consists of the drug companies supplying the drugs, the investigators and their support staff conducting the actual research, the ethics committee and institutional review board. Both groups are the only ones necessary for any drug clinical trial to be completed successfully besides the oversight from the FDA. Once the study or clinical trial is completed, the results are collated and analyzed and organized for presentation to the regulatory agencies and perhaps for publication in a journal. They can then submit their results to these regulatory agencies for approval for the indications the drug was tested for. That's the typical situation. Most of the HCQ clinical trials are however not typical because besides the giver and recipient groups, there are "special interest groups". These groups either have an axe to grind, something to gain that is being threatened, or a determination to promote something other than what is best for the patient. The whole point of a clinical trial is to provide a patient with an option in the absence of none, a better option which may mean something inexpensive, safer, familiar, affordable, available, something perhaps life saving, relatively inexpensive, affordable and available at the lowest possible production costs in the safest possible dose.

Several of the studies reviewed earlier and the way these studies were done should tell you not to trust what you read or hear about clinical trials or "scientific evidence" until you have methodically examined the details of the study yourself. In this chapter I am going to show you a clinical trial design that could have been used for evaluating the efficacy of HCQ in Covid-19. You'll be able to draw conclusions about the design feasibility and outcomes intelligently.

Lastly, I'd like to provide a classification of doctors and healthcare professionals based on their response to Covid-19 and on the direct or indirect interactions I have had with them or their knowledge. With respect to Covid-19, there are two types of health care professionals, those that know what they need to know about this pandemic and those that don't know what they need to know. These two major groups are further subdivided based on their willingness to know what they don't, those who are just plain petrified and frozen and those that just don't care.

Group 1 MD's – (Don't Know Covid)
   a. Don't know and scared
   b. Don't know and don't care
   c. Don't know but care to know
   d. Don't know but care about patients not dying or suffering

Group 2 MD's – (Know Covid and HCQ)
   a. Know but scared
   b. Know and don't care because of politics
   c. Know and don't care about patients dying
   d. Know and care about patients but confused about what to do
   e. Know and only care about making money and paying bills
   f. Know but not all they need to know
   g. Know and doing something to change everything

If you belong to Groups 1a, 1c, 1d, 2a, 2d, 2f, then get the information you need by creating the time and researching independently or and

163

colleagues good at interpreting these studies. Create the time. I wrote this book based on information that is out there without paying for a single piece of research. Find out what others are doing to help their Covid-19 patients, and if you've read this far, you do have a lot of helpful information you can now put to use. Continue learning and adopt a student-for-life mentality. I read voraciously. And it has helped save my patients on few occasions. So find empowerment by connecting with others in the profession who know what they're doing.

For those in 1b, it's hard to figure out why you chose the healthcare profession. Despite our varying personalities, the number one trait that drove us into the healthcare profession is that we care, a lot.

Group 2c and 2e are the ones easily approached by Dr. Frank Gambini and Boris Cheyenko to lower the bar of humanity even further. They don't care about anyone other than themselves. They may be highly skilled, brilliant and experienced, but the only thing that matters to them is their reputation, and what they want. They will not hesitate to compromise on their beliefs as long as there is something in it for them. You might say these are the Judases of the healthcare profession. They will kill if they have to, as long as it can be done subtly where no one can see them, because they have bills to pay; alimony, child support, big house, expensive cars, things that add nothing of value to you as a person. These group is quite diverse in their tastes and motives and it's uncertain what they might be willing to do just to get money or how much they delight in human suffering, power or control. You can see the different categories of healthcare professionals in your real life and in the authors of some of the research papers mentioned earlier in this book. To group 2f belong those doctors that know just a little about Covid-19 but not enough of what they need to know and are often found in the media saying "it's not been proven" or "we need randomized double blinded, placebo controlled trials to show that HCQ really works" or "HCQ is ineffective in Covid-19". Having read this far, what is the likelihood that you've heard, seen or met such a doctor? Perhaps you've even been diagnosed with Covid-19 and your scared healthcare provider didn't know what to do for you. You can see why doctors in all these categories behave differently about Covid-19, even the ones you thought were quite knowledgeable before Covid-19.

Let's now look at a concept for designing truly useful efficacy clinical trials for HCQ. We'll start by looking at two scenarios. The first scenario is one in which a scientific breakthrough has revealed that there are five different types of Covid-19 patients, A, B, C, D and E. Each of these five groups of patients will respond to a different drug and the drug will be 100% curative. Four drugs, ARx, BRx, CRx, and DRx have been found to cure Covid-19 groups A, B, C, and D respectively with 100% efficacy if given at the right time. So we now need to develop a fifth drug for group E patients because the drugs for groups A through D have only 20% maximum efficacy in group E Covid-19 patients.

In the second scenario, four drugs, one new one and three others already approved by CDA (Cooking and Drug Administration) for other conditions, were found to be effective in preliminary studies. Your clinic with four others, have been selected to conduct clinical trials. Each of you will study only one drug and each drug already has an approved safety profile. A ballot was drawn for all five of you and you end up with drug E. You win the contest. Let's look at how your clinical trial was designed.

First research question:
Is drug ERx effective in Group E Covid-19 patients?

You decide you will design a clinical trial for efficacy, the details of which will be ironed out later. Before doing that however you must figure out what the next question should be. According to Dr. Rita Popat, Stanford University Clinical Associate Professor of Epidemiology, Health Research and Policy, that next research question should be

Will a randomized double-blinded placebo controlled study answer this question?

Since the onset of the Covid-19 pandemic, multiple studies have been published based on well thought out designs to measure the efficacy of HCQ. Some of these studies have however shown avoidable weaknesses and flaws, especially those using toxic doses of HCQ to remind us of Auschwitz and Tuskegee. The investigators of the RECOVERY study carefully removed the toxic dosages of HCQ they initially published on their web pages. May be the deletion of HCQ was an oversight but it disappeared from page 22 of the same document. Also, the eminent professors commenting on the RECOVERY study carefully overlooked the toxic doses of HCQ and that included a Professor of pharmacoepidemiology at the London School of Tropical Medicine and Hygiene. You might need a little help understanding the role a Professor of pharmacoepidemiology at the famous London School plays in chloroquine and hydroxychloroquine prescriptions in the malaria

165

The HCQ Debate, Caxton Opere, MD

infested developing countries around the world. Such a professor of tropical medicine knows at least one drug dosage so well and that drug is chloroquine and its analog, hydroxychloroquine. These professors train doctors and healthcare workers around the world on how to manage several tropical and infectious diseases. The clinical efficacy and safety of any hated drug like hydroxychloroquine can be prospectively designed so it fails safety and efficacy trials. An oncologist colleague looking at the Brazilian study came to the conclusion that the study was designed so HCQ could fail. A cursory glance at the methodology section may fail to reveal this plot. You have to know how to thoroughly evaluate journal articles of importance and draw your own conclusions regardless of what the conclusion in the abstract section states.

So in designing safety and efficacy trials for Group E Covid-19 patients, toxic dosing must be avoided. ER'x's standard dosing is known. Patients will be recruited who have been either exposed within 24 hours for the prophylactic arm, and these exposed with symptoms no more than 48 hours will be tested and if positive started on the early treated arm. Since we now know that about 80% have minimal or no symptoms, about 15% get hospitalized and roughly 5% become critically ill enough to be admitted to the ICU, asymptomatic patients will also be included if they are Covid-19 positive. Since mortality is quite high and approved drugs are already available, a randomized double-blinded placebo controlled study will be unethical. Treatment will be randomized and double-blinded but it cannot be placebo-controlled. We cannot expect to recruit enough patients into the study if their family member died of Covid-19 and they are told they may not get the effective treatment. Patients come to the clinic or hospital to get treated not to be guinea pigs for Covid-19 experiments. We want to know if there is a specific group of Covid-19 patients in which E is effective and those in which it will not be effective. Crossovers, drop ins and dropout will be expected and will be expected and be handled according to protocol.

Primary Outcomes: Well-defined objective parameters of efficacy for outpatients, in-patients and ICU patients such as improvements in viral clearance, pH, pO2, lactic acid, reduced need for oxygen supplementation, extubation without re-intubation will be used. Subjective primary outcomes that include symptom resolution, discharge will also be determined. Death is a crude primary outcome and will be recorded with specific cause of death as Covid-19 patients may die of non-Covid causes.

Objective markers of disease: Objective markers of disease and disease severity will be used such as cytokine levels, ferritin as well as degree of hypoxia

Surrogate markers of disease: Measured day 3, 7 and 14 as objective markers of illness on specific days.
It'll be important to measure at least one surrogate marker such as cytokine levels of severity during randomization. This will help us better understand several things such as

1. Correlations between surrogate markers and illness severity at randomization
2. Correlations between surrogate markers and disease progression
3. If there is a correlation between the surrogate marker and drug efficacy. Do objective measures of surrogate marker correlate well with improvement or decline while on treatment? Do sicker patients respond better to the drug or is it only mildly ill patients that respond
4. What do surrogate markers tell us about timing of therapy in order to better understand stage-drug-disease interactions
5. What is the best timing for this maximal benefit to be obtained
6. Do surrogate markers correlate with patient outcomes such as death

Epidemiological markers: Are there any epidemiological markers that can reveal efficacy differences based on age, Socio-economic status

Biological markers: Comorbidities, Sex, Genetics. Any other abnormal laboratory findings found on routine tests will be documented for later review.

Crossover will be allowed and drop-in and dropouts accounted for in the final analysis. Use of surrogate markers will be a step forward in eliminating subjective bias that weakens the data fidelity. Researchers should have carefully addressed these issues before commencing their study. If they had, most of the problems practitioners now have, and the confusion about how to treat Covid-19 patients, will not exist at this point of the pandemic. Was it an intentional oversight? We may never know.

Blinding

The HCQ Debate, Caxton Opere, MD

Failure to blind means your biases will be used to redirect the study towards whatever outcome you desire. So every open labeled studied is of the lowest quality. Brazilian Coalition was an open label study. The study will be triple or quadruple double blinded. Treating physicians, patients, statisticians, and everyone participating will not know who is taking what.

You're probably dealing with one of the greatest medical cover-ups in the history of benevolent medicine in the face of a deadly pandemic. Someone should be held responsible. I know you can find so much proof showing that HCQ works and many developing countries continue to report success with basic drugs such as HCQ combined with zinc, quercetin, azithromycin, vitamin C and D as well as simpler remedies such as ginger in very mild or recently exposed Covid-19 cases. Whatever your thoughts, be assured that information that could have helped or prevented the deaths and illness in millions around the world from Covid-19 seems to have been intentionally withheld and then toxic drug doses were administered to clinical trial subjects to make one of the most effective drugs for Covid-19 look like the most dangerous drug on the planet despite its 65-year excellent safety profile.

33

A Billionaire's Little Secret

George Sachs is a philanthropist billionaire who has donated so many billions to India and South America. Having studied the wealthy in sufficient depth over the last two decades and doing his Master's thesis on the wealthy, Bill Blass, a best-selling author and Podcaster, decides to look into this unusual degree of generosity by a man who was came from a very wealthy family. His motivation for this depth of generosity just didn't make sense to Bill. George Sachs' parents were millionaires but George Sachs is a multibillionaire worth a few hundred billion, and no one really knows how much he is worth. Bill did finally get the interview opportunity. George offered to grant him the interview on one condition, that Bill would fly down to meet him in London Luton Airport and fly with George to Paris on a Gulfstream. When Bill asked George on arrival in Paris when they would meet for the interview, George replied with a smile that Bill had twenty minutes starting right then. But Bill was prepared and the single most important question was why was George giving away all that money to people that can't pay him back? George's reply was "billionaires play for the long haul". He answered a few more questions but the one that Bill couldn't get off his mind as he walked into the *Louvre* the next morning was the phrase "billionaires play for the long haul". In deep thought, Bill knew the clue to George's generosity was hidden in that answer, but he couldn't figure it out. When he arrived back in New Jersey, Monday evening, he called Bruno Galli, a billionaire he had interviewed for his wealth thesis, and had taken Bill like a son. Bruno was the one that had inspired him to do a wealth thesis, a project that eventually got him on the New York Times Bestseller list. Bruno smiled as they sat down at the recently reopened café since the lockdown and explained the real George Sachs to Bill Blass. "Playing for the long haul", Bruno said meant George was playing to gain the trust of not only the governments of those developing countries, but the people there too. They all love and trust George, at least most of them. George was playing for high stakes, for trillions, and he has donated millions while waiting patiently until this pandemic. With the corona vaccine George's company was working on, and the RFID (radio frequency identity) chip that governments all over the world will be buying from him in about five months, shortly after the US Presidential election. "George Sachs has 7 billion potential customers that will be paying him at least one thousand dollars a piece, directly or indirectly for the Covid-19 drug, Covid-19 vaccine, the RFID chip and by people from all over the world," Bruno whispered silently, as he asked the barrister for the check.

One question that may be lingering in your mind after examining all this material is why? Why would Professors of medicine engage in this level of complicity that has led to the death of so many around the world? Could it be money, power, a sense of superiority over others, a sadistic tendency to watch people die, or something more sinister? You be the judge. My prayer is that this book gets into the hands of men and women who know right from wrong and can influence the laws of their land to prevail in bringing those responsible to justice.

34

Bad News from Your Last Flight

Imagine you flew to Hawaii on vacation and just came back last night. Early this morning at about 7am, you receive a call from the airline and the caller alerts you that the call was for contact tracing purposes because one of the passengers, precisely the one sitting next to you on the plane, had just died of Covid-19. They were calling to inform you so you could go see your doctor. Without HCQ, the fear that will plague you for the next few hours or weeks can be horrifying. Yet HCQ can provide the necessary safe guard and peace of mind by prophylactic use to put your mind at ease. Yet those who are designing studies to make it look as if HCQ is inefficient in prophylaxis or early treatment are not brought to justice. They should be, because they are perpetuating fear and making sure the drug is not used when it can be most effective, invariably increasing the incidence of new infections and eventually increased number of deaths. It's either they don't care, they've been bought, or they're caught up on methodology that they are ignoring the realities of clinical medicine. No one wants to be a guinea pig and die while on a placebo. While HCQ works and many healthcare professionals attest to its efficacy, they are often shooed because of lack of RCT's. There will not be any RCT's for HCQ as it is unethical. Giving the patient who just got off the plane HCQ with or without azithromycin would be the best thing to do for this patient, you! But if you do not understand the far-reaching effects of Big Pharma, look at the CDC website. It's as if the scientists that drew up the information on Covid-19 either cannot read the journals properly, which indeed would be a shame, and is probably unlikely, or because they've probably been bought or threatened.

Around the rest of the world, where there is no hatred of HCQ, and where people just want to get better without the influence of lobbyists, HCQ works.

Let's look outside our politically divided America for information about hydroxychloroquine:

What do experts in Belgium & Bahrain say?

https://justthenews.com/politics-policy/coronavirus/bahrain-

The HCQ Debate, Caxton Opere, MD

hydroxychloroquine-success-response-covid-19

How about Brazil?

https://riotimesonline.com/brazil-news/miscellaneous/early-hydroxychloroquine-use-reduced-deaths-by-60-percent-says-prevent-senior/

What's happening in Costa Rica?

https://surfguardcr.com/local-news/costa-rica/costa-rica-prescribing-hydroxychloroquine-for-covid-19-patients

What do experts in India say?

https://timesofindia.indiatimes.com/india/hydroxychloroquine-should-be-used-as-prophylaxis-not-as-treatment-for-covid-19-icmr/articleshow/75098629.cms

How about Italy?
(https://www.3ccorp.net/2020/04/30/media-lied-people-died-italian-study-finds-incredible-prophylaxis-results-for-patients-on-hydroxychloroquine/)

Morocco, because it is "independent of pharmaceuticals":
(https://www.moroccoworldnews.com/2020/05/301362/french-politician-morocco-far-superior-to-france-in-covid-19-response/)

How about Senegal?

https://redandblackonline.com/senegal-touts-the-effects-of-chloroquine-supporting-figures/

How about South Korea--one of the most successful cases?

https://www.upi.com/Top_News/World-News/2020/03/12/South-Korea-experts-recommend-anti-HIV-anti-malaria-drugs-for-COVID-19/6961584012321/

What is Turkey reporting?

https://www.cbsnews.com/news/hydroxychloroquine-coronavirus-covid-19-treatment-turkey/

What is the United Arab Emirates doing?
(https://english.alarabiya.net/en/coronavirus/2020/04/12/Coronaviru
s-UAE-says-it-is-successfully-treating-patients-with-
hydroxychloroquine)

Algeria
(http://www.algerianembassy.org/press/covid-19-l-algerie-a-adopte-
une-strategie-lui-permettant-de-maitriser-la-situation.html)

What of the Chinese & French studies?

https://live.healthday.com/hydroxychloroquine-shorten-recovery-time-
covid-19-2645652660.html?rebelltitem=1#rebelltitem1

https://techstartups.com/2020/04/06/french-researcher-dr-didier-
raoult-has-now-treated-1000-coronavirus-patient-with-99-3-success-rate/

What do all these stories and testimonies tell us about HCQ? Simply
that the politicization of HCQ intentionally or otherwise has cost many
Americans their lives and livelihoods. It's time for us as doctors to wake
up and read the same journals and sift through the lies we've all
believed.

The HCQ Debate, Caxton Opere, MD

A New Gold Standard for Clinical Trials:

Prospective, randomized, double-blinded, placebo controlled where ethically acceptable, without administration of toxic doses of study drug(s), void of any conflict of interest, with proper interpretation of study data and genuine implications for improvement of human health conditions.

Moving forward, if you want to classify clinical trials in terms of real quality, this table should help you.

Scoring Standards for Clinical Human Research

Standard	*P=4 R=3 Cs=2 Cr=1	Random ized	Double-blinded	Place bo-contro lled	Toxic or lethal drug Doses	Proper Conclusion	Conflict of interest-political, $$, or by association	Points
Platinum	P	+	+	+	No	+	No	10
Diamond	P	+	+	+	No	+	No	10
Gold	P	+	+	+	+/-	+	No	9
Silver	R	+	+	+	No	+	Yes	5
Bronze	P	+	+	+	No	No	Yes	4
Iron	R	+	+	+	+	No	Yes	1
Woods	Cs	+	-	-	No	No	Yes	0
Stone	Cs	-	-	-	No	No	Yes	-1
Plastic	Cr	-	-	-	No	No	Yes	-2

*Prospective, P=4; Retrospective, R=3; Case studies, Cs=2; Case report, Cr=1.
Conflict of interest = -3 points; Improper conclusion = -1; toxic lethal doses = -1(+/- =0,

As you can see from RECOVERY, SOLIDARITY, COALITION, DisCoveRy and many others, these were substandard HCQ studies that do not improve the human health condition and may have cost many innocent victims their lives. Data was designed to lie, inconclusive and weak and many of the authors even admit that their studies did not benefit mankind. It's time for a change. Clinical investigators in human research MUST be held to higher human standards regardless of informed consent. When it can be deciphered that toxic doses of medications have been administered to unsuspecting subjects, or regular doses of poisonous substances such as plutonium given to Ebb Cade on March 24, 1945, justice ought to be served. Ebb Cade, an African American truck driver, had sustained multiple fractures in an accident. Researchers thought he was going to die from the accident, so they started experimenting on him for months. One day, they found out he was gone. He had healed well enough to plot his escape from the torture lab. His teeth were pulled and he was injected with radioactive material for about 6 months. Too many horrid accounts have been documented over the last 8 decades of medical experiments on humans unaware of the fact they were been exposed or injected with dangerous substances.

When you attack those supporting the use of hydroxychloroquine while patients using it with or without zinc are getting treated and cured, recognize that your behavior reflects either one of ignorance or recklessness. You became part of the problem of human abuse propagated in the name of "science" of which the Nazi's were a great participant. Many patients should not have died if given an opportunity to start HCQ early, and asides from the vaccine, which I suspect will not be protective or safe if released this early, there is nothing really available to treat Covid-19 that the NIH or CDC wants to agree with till we find a better cure. So choose your side well in the debate because it's more than HCQ at stake, it's the freedom of mankind at stake. When Karen Whitsett, a Black Democrat in Michigan thanked the US President for his actions with respect to Covid-19, the 13th Congressional District of the Democratic Party descended on her with fangs, trying to destroy her. That's what may happen to you very soon in what is supposed to be a free country. There will be another attempted lockdown that can only be foiled by the truth that sets men free and if you have an opportunity to make a real difference, make that difference regardless of your political leanings. Black iatraphobia, fear or of medical care, may be fueling the HCQ debate, but as you can see already, that same phobia is going to manifest once the Covid-19 vaccine finally arrives.

Instead of focusing on when to use HCQ and who will benefit the most from its use, millions of dollars are been spent trying to prove HCQ doesn't work. That's not scientific. It's insanity. But if the goal is to make trillions, good try. There are several groups of doctors and patients in and outside the United States who have had firsthand experience of the benefits of HCQ in the treatment of Covid-19. They are unperturbed by

The HCQ Debate, Caxton Opere, MD

the misleading research news and drama and continue to get great success with HCQ despite the media misinformation. The practitioners are treating the patients successfully and Gambini therefore extended his tentacles to have the pharmacists refuse to fill prescriptions in so many States in the country. These are the same pharmacists that allowed an opioid epidemic and opioid deaths to reach crisis levels by filling too many narcotic prescriptions for the same patient. They now want to prevent doctors from prescribing the only real early treatment for Covid-19 patients, a 5 to 7-day course of HCQ. I'm not sure pharmacists get sued for negligence but if they do, it'll be a very rare thing. Unfortunately, there may soon be a rise in lawsuits against pharmacists that refused to fill HCQ prescriptions for patients that eventually die for lack of early treatment. When that happens, it may signify that a previously unheard of professional disaster, tsunami-like in proportion, will descend on the safe profession of pharmacy. Doctors that have equally felt berated and degraded by pharmacists after prescribing the drug could also start reporting grievances creating another line of firing at pharmacists negligent in their duty by failing to fill these prescriptions. It could get very ugly very quickly, if a patient that could have survived dies for not getting a needed script and it becomes clear that the research against HCQ in early treatment was all a fraud.

Why would any pharmacist want to be in the midst of such nonsense? All the pharmacists that I know and have spoken with personally know the value of HCQ in the treatment of early Covid-19 infection. A house divided against itself cannot stand, and some pharmacists for whatever reason may bring their own house down. You don't like a President saying a drug works, so what? Is that the reason to not give the drug to those who might benefit from it and by benefit we mean reduced likelihood of worsening illness, need for hospitalization, mechanical ventilation or death. The first item on the Cheyenko plan was to attach HCQ to someone disliked by many, and whether you believe it or not, HCQ has been firmly attached to President Donald Trump. Everyone around the world knows this. He says it works, admits to using it, but very few understand the crafty nature of those working the Cheyenko plan behind the scenes.

HCQ vs. Big Pharma, David vs. Goliath?

Few people are aware of the $233 million contributed by Big Pharma annually into the hands of senatorial and presidential candidates and elections. Even if we don't like or trust politicians, there is one group of individuals or institutions that we trust, professors and academic medical centers. The integrity of some papers published in the *New England Journal of Medicine* is now in question for any reasonable physician that reads journals thoroughly. According to a November 24, 2012 *Washington Post* article by Peter Whoriskey, the NEJM published 73 articles on new drugs of which 60 were funded by a pharmaceutical company, 50 co-written by a drug company employee. One of those drugs was Avandia for the treatment of diabetes, a drug that was later found to be responsible for more than 80,000 heart attacks according to the FDA. More recently, the behavior of some English Professors towards the RECOVERY study in England lends suspicion to how much tainted academic medicine is today. If politicians can be lobbied, how much more academic medicine! Peter Whoriskey stated that while the NIH spent $31 billion on research in 2011, Big Pharma spent a whopping $39 billion! So if we think it's only politicians that bow to Big Pharma, academic professors may have to bow even lower. Do academic centers have an obligation to the people or to Big Pharma? While we expect the highest degree of intellectual material and research from academic medical centers, it seems that since the Covid-19 pandemic started, there is no guarantee that a professor of medicine will not lie if there is enough incentive from a pharmaceutical company to do so. And if one professor can lie, what stops an entire department or even prestigious medical institution from deceiving the world in order to profit? Avandia was recalled, multiple lawsuits followed, yet in the midst of the unfolding tragedy about Avandia, a group of doctors *(Home et., al N Engl J Med 2007; 357:28-38)*, wrote an article stating Avandia was associated with an increase in heart failure but not heart attacks in their study of 4447 patients, but to what effect? To try and cover up the 80,000 plus heart attacks?

The motives for attacking HCQ from all flanks should be obvious to you by now. It's about just one thing, money, profit, trillions. You see, the reason it is clear that Big Pharma is behind the attacks on HCQ is that they are the only ones that profit if HCQ does not work. Have you ever heard of a situation where patients are dying and doctors say a drug works to save lives and prevent hospitalization, and some other doctors suddenly take another cohort and try to prove that the drug doesn't work? Never. That's not science. Science will try to understand why HCQ worked in my patients (early Covid-19) but not in Dr. Higginbotham's patients (late Covid-19). Science would try to understand and stratify in whom HCQ will work and in whom it wouldn't work. Nevertheless, the FDA, CDC and NIH strongly recommend against the use of HCQ under any circumstances except in clinical trials. That's bad science, motivated by Big Pharma's influence, and an attack on the practice of medicine. Why bother using it in clinical trials alone if it isn't effective in other circumstances? The August 27, 2020 recommendations by the NIH says

- *The COVID-19 Treatment Guidelines Panel (the Panel) recommends against the use of any agents for SARS-CoV-2 pre-exposure prophylaxis (PrEP), except in clinical trials (AIII).*
- *The Panel recommends against the use of any agents for SARS-CoV-2 post-exposure prophylaxis (PEP), except in a clinical trial. (AIII).*

Guess who pays for most clinical trials? Big Pharma! Are you surprised that even the NIH has ceded the proper practice of medicine to clinical trials, as if doctors were trained to do clinical trials rather than take care of patients. Most doctors who care for patients practice medicine with intention and most clinics and hospitals and are not research centers. Clinical trials have different moving arms and if clinical trials are the only place to use HCQ, it's so that the "experts" can manipulate anything they want and nullify HCQ treatment effects through statistical manipulations. If 300 confirmed Covid-19 positive patients get treated in a clinic with HCQ and their symptoms resolved completely with a negative Covid-19 test 5 days later, you can't argue with that result. Even if it was 270 of them that got cured, you still can't argue with a 90% success. But put the same 300 patients in a clinical trial, and then hire experts to distort the truth in order to make HCQ look ineffective and you'd be amazed at what statisticians can do. So insisting that HCQ not be given outside the hospital except in clinical trials is a Gambini method. They're trying to leave the window open for possible use of HCQ in case they can't find a drug that works or an effective vaccine, but at the same time, they're saying no one should use HCQ, until they find a drug that works and costs a fortune. Such pitiful arrogance! If people are dying, why not create helpful guidelines and encourage doctors to prescribe HCQ rather than watch patients get hospitalized and critically ill? If the NIH, FDA and CDC really cared about the people dying, they would come up with something useful like:

TO ALL PHYSICIANS PRESCRIBING HCQ TO COVID-19 PATIENTS:

"We strongly recommend against the use of HCQ but since you intend to prescribe it and it may have some benefit at the early stages of infection, you might as well get some important guidelines as we also want the best for the American people and do not want those who could potentially benefit from HCQ to die if in fact it is effective in some Covid-19 patients"

The CDC and NIH I used to know back then would then go ahead and share some useful information with doctors to help patients in the outpatient setting if in fact "HCQ works". You now know that in the absence of distorted reporting in scientific journals, the CDC, FDA and NIH should have reported the clinically and pharmacologically predicted efficacy of HCQ and the following:

1. Give HCQ only after obtaining Covid-19 test samples in symptomatic patients
2. Do not give Azithromycin with HCQ to patients over the age of X, Y or Z unless you perform an EKG.
3. Both Azithromycin and HCQ have long half lives and so it is possible that one or two doses of Azithromycin may be enough to perform the stereotactic blocking at the molecular level to hinder attachment of the virus to the QFN-triad on SARS-CoV-2
4. If you are the only doctor in your practice, stick to only one regimen so that when your data is later analyzed, we can determine the most effective regimen from pooling data from other centers. If you choose two different regimens, give each regimen a name like A or B, I or II, so that on retrieving your data for analysis later, you can help the CDC and NIH identify the most effective regimen
5. If you are part of a group of physicians with different regimens for HCQ, formalize your regimen like a standing order so that each regimen has a specific name or label and can be compared with others in your practice
6. Send every hypoxic patient to the hospital no matter how confident you are about HCQ
7. Get your suspicious patients tested immediately and tell them to start HCQ immediately
8. Revive any other useful information from the EUA and least

Even if this would save only 5 percent of the over 200,000 patients that have died, that would have been at least an additional 10,000 lives saved early and perhaps never getting hospitalized. The number is likely to be

The HCQ Debate, Caxton Opere, MD

much higher if you ask the right pharmacoepidemiologists. It makes no sense to tell doctors not to practice medicine and practice research instead! I didn't swear to research but to care for patients. As you can see, not only is it costing more lives to practice research, researchers are manipulating data and conclusions to fit a narrative that enables Big Pharma to then try and make the most profit at the cost of human lives. Think about how many trillions Big Pharma is trying to make. Then think about how many trillions of dollars have equally been lost from the pandemic in the United States alone. It's an ecosystem that drains away trillions of dollars from the economy and then siphons several trillions of dollars more into one entity, Big Pharma. The numbers will probably approximate each other but I'll leave that to economists. What should be done instead of telling doctors not to prescribe HCQ is to admit it works in some patients, early during the course of the illness, perhaps only in a few cases, or maybe in a lot more (early cases) and then research HCQ regimens that are effective in PrEP, PEP and early treatment. Then let doctors use these regimens judiciously. Instead we get these published journal articles revealing the tainted system of academic medical research and health policy formulation. Big Pharma already knows HCQ works and that it would disrupt the insane profit they hope to make and they are going to make sure that never happens.

The following HCQ regimens are suggested to the US government so interested clinicians as well as researchers can find efficacy and safety profiles for HCQ in Covid-19. None of them exceed the 2.4g in the original and revoked EUA for HCQ:

A. HCQ EARLY TREATMENT REGIMENS TO RESEARCH FURTHER
400mg twice daily on day 1; 400mg daily days 2-5 =2.4g
400mg twice daily on days 1 & 2; 400mg daily days 3 & 4 =2.4g
400mg twice daily x 3 days = 2.4g
400mg twice daily on day 1; 400mg daily days 2-4 = 2g
Day 1, 400mg twice daily; day 2, 400mg in the morning 200mg at night; day 3, 200mg twice a day; day 4, 200mg once = 2g

With zinc and with or without azithromycin.

B. HCQ POST-EXPOSURE PROPHYLAXIS
400mg twice daily on day 1; 400mg daily days 2-5 = 2.4g
400mg twice daily on days 1 & 2; 400mg daily days 3 & 4 =2.4g
400mg twice daily x 3 days = 2.4g
400mg twice daily on day 1; 400mg daily days 2-4 = 2g
Day 1 400mg twice daily; day 2, 400mg in the morning 200mg at night; day 3, 200mg twice a day; day 200mg once = 2g

C. HCQ PRE-EXPOSURE PROPHYLAXIS
200mg every two weeks
200mg every week
400mg every two weeks
400mg every 4 weeks
With or without zinc and with other adjuncts like vitamin C or D.
Some hospitals, provide their ER doctors azithromycin as well as HCQ and have had 100% efficacy!

As you probably are aware, there are doctors prescribing HCQ for pre-exposure prophylaxis, and to a very large group of patients for that matter, millions of them. Before your rush off to the FDA to report these doctors, they are using it for patients diagnosed with rheumatoid arthritis (RA) and systemic lupus (SLE), rheumatological conditions that potentially quadruple the risk of Covid-19. Yet the incidence of Covid-19 in patients with RA and SLE taking HCQ is far lower than expected in several studies. *(Ferreira et al, 2020)*.

Big Pharma lives off of the pain of individuals even when they're not in a crisis situation. So I'm almost certain they now feel it's their right to not let this pandemic "go to waste". They've donated billions and they want a payback in trillions. The only real stumbling block to these trillions are high-ranking individuals in academic medicine and health policy making officials already eating from the palm of their hands. These officials will do anything to help their Big brother, Big Pharma.

Except they work for Gabini, any scientist worth his weight will NEVER say HCQ is ineffective in Covid-19 after reading the journals shared in this book. The irony of it is that these are the same journals used to denounce HCQ because we refused to read the entire papers. Simply listening to CNN journalists quoting the most trusted medical journal in the world in its widest margin of error, without actually reading the article themselves, has caught many doctors off guard. I can understand the plight of those that don't know how to read research articles, but a seasoned doctor saying HCQ doesn't work is simply a show of ignorance contributes to the US Covid-19 death rates. You might find some academics cockily denying financial conflict of interest at the end of their research articles or comments against HCQ. How many of the grants their department or University receives annually come from Big Pharma in and outside the United States? Probably a substantial amount! I am not opposed to profit and I have a great delight in seeing every business prosper, Big Pharma inclusive, but to deceive, taint the most trusted medical professionals in academic institutions and those with excellent

The HCQ Debate, Caxton Opere, MD

academic credentials, in other to perpetuate a lie that destroys so many jobs, get so many killed, and sweep in profits like a vulture, is not good business, it's economic sabotage. If in fact it can be proven, then the culprits should be brought to justice. The pain in my heart as I've watched the number of deaths soar during this pandemic is nothing short of anguishing. I'm even more angered by the journalists who think they know so much about Covid-19, mocking doctors who know exactly what they're doing by recommending or prescribing HCQ. Journalists that cannot read the truth hiding in plain sight in the journals they are quoting as randomized controlled studies. How can you quote a randomized controlled "open label" study as authoritative and then proceed to insult another doctor about his decision to recommend HCQ when these "randomized controlled" reek of flaws? Beats me.

HCQ vs. Big Pharma, David vs. Goliath, Pennies vs. Trillions

According to wellrx.com, 60 tablets of generic hydroxychloroquine costs $19.39 at HEB Pharmacy and $19.44 at Kroger, $23.06 at Costco, $29.77 at Walmart pharmacy. The regimens listed earlier used a maximum of 12 pills per person or less. So for the 2.4g regimens, these 60 pills will treat 5 people. Which means the cost of HCQ treatment per person will be less than $5. In addition "if HCQ is effective in Covid-19" when started early, then the cost, sorrow and pains of hospitalization will be eliminated completely. What does Big Pharma have to offer? Remdesivir? It not only comes at a nice price of about $3200 per treatment, the system has been well orchestrated such that by the time the patient requires it, they are so sick they have to be hospitalized. So the cost of using remdesivir is not just $3,200 but additional hospitalization costs that include medications, resources and adjuncts such as lab tests. For the sake of simplicity however, let's limit the contrast between using HCQ early to Remdesivir just to drug prices. You are aware that hospitalization costs for severely ill and even fairly healthy patients can be quite substantial. According to www.healthcarefinancenews.com, the cost for uninsured Covid-19 patients could be as high as $73,000 or as low as $17,094 for the insured. All because government agencies like the NIH and CDC release updates that intimidate doctors already at risk of litigation from prescribing HCQ. If HCQ "was effective in Covid-19", it would $5 per prescription. Contrast this with either $3200 for a regimen of Remdesivir, $17,094 or the total cost of caring for a hospitalized Covid-19 patient. Either way you do the math, $3,200 divided by 5 is over 640 times the cost of HCQ and $17,094 divided by 5 is 3,418 times the cost of HCQ. It's the government that's allowed this to go on, and the government that has the power to stop this. Why be a stumbling block to the most effective treatment in the early stages of Covid-19 infection? It's about the profit, and in this case, playing on people's fears – fear of death, fear of getting sued, fear of being wrong. In most instances, once HCQ is started, the patients never get to the hospital. That's what the CDC is supposed to help with specific treatment strategies not send us to the NIH website with updates reeking of Big Pharma influence.

As you could see from the shoddily designed clinical trials bent on disproving the use of HCQ, you need to be sure you don't become a victim of fatally misguided "science and data" robots who really don't care who dies as long as they get paid or as long as they feel they have a political axe to grind. What's amazing is that while you're joining the band wagon, you can't be absolutely certain that the people denouncing HCQ in public don't have a stash of HCQ and are using it for prophylaxis and treatment of their family members regularly. I care about people and that's what drove me to medicine and kept me there and if that's why you read this far, you ought to admit that something dangerously fraudulent has taken place in the US in the last 10 months

The unified scientific incoherence between researchers, the FDA, NIH, CDC, academic medicine, liberal journalists and the published papers they are misinterpreting leaves me with one question for you:

Considering the trillions of dollars of potential profit Big Pharma hopes to make from this pandemic, do you think is there is an effort to undermine the efficacy of hydroxychloroquine in Covid-19 infections and why?

Hopefully, after reading this book, your attitude to the most trusted research papers will skepticism.

The HCQ Debate, Caxton Opere, MD

AUTHOR'S TRAILER: APPENDIX and SCRATCH PAD

When writing, authors usually throw away a lot of good material. I decided to let you in on valuable stuff that didn't make the cut. So this is a little bit of scrap that would not have made it inside the book. It's valuable material that didn't quite fit the flow of the book, a behind the scenes trailer equivalent. Enjoy.

SAFE HYDROXYCHLOROQUINE REGIMENS FOR OUTPATIENT TREATMENT

Caution in the use of Azithromycin with HCQ due to QT prolongation. By caution it means consult with a primary care doctor if these drugs are available over the counter where you live. Get an EKG and have the intervals measured and recorded on your chart. Get another EKG within 24 hours and perhaps 48 hours after starting treatment with both drugs.

CASIS OUTPATIENT
HCQ
Day 1: 400mg bid x 1 day (12 hours apart)
Day 2-5: 400mg daily x 4 more days
*Azithromycin: 500mg day 1 only in those at risk for QT prolongation but no QT prolongation
ZnSO4 220mg daily
Vitamin C 500mg daily
Vitamin D3 2000U daily
Thiamine 200mg daily

The CASIS outpatient regimen is given with or without azithromycin, depending on the risk for arrhythmia based on past history, current presentation, cytokine levels and abnormal EKG and ability to get a repeat EKG in 24 hours after starting treatment. **A QRS duration of less than 100ms makes lethal toxicity from cardiac arrhythmia or abnormal QT prolongation unlikely.** (Watson et al. 2020.) *The QT interval may change after starting azithromycin with HCQ and a repeat EKG may be needed particularly if initial EKG showed any abnormality, if the patient is on multiple drugs that can prolong QT, if the patient is hypertensive, or if the patient has other comorbidities that increase the risk of sudden cardiac death such as morbid obesity, sleep apnea, prior arrhythmias, coronary artery disease, diabetes, peripheral vascular disease, prior stroke.*

NON-HCQ COVID-19 REGIMENS
Since the ultimate mechanism by which Covid-19 makes people sick requires replication and zinc can inhibit the enzyme for replication RdRp, you may treat Covid-19 without HCQ. Give a zing ionophore and be sure to start early following exposure to SARS-CoV-2 and the onset of symptoms.

ZnSO4 220mg daily x 7 days
Quercetin 500mg twice daily x 7 days
Vitamin C 1g twice daily x 7 days
Vitamin D3 3000U daily x 7 days
Thiamine 200mg daily x 7 days

A DANGEROUS DIALOGUE

An argument ensued between the hospital medical director and a newly hired doctor. The doctor refused to recommend any treatment for a sick admitted Covid-19 patient. The nursing director called the medical director because as there were no written orders for the patient and the patient's family had been expecting something to be done by the eight hours they had been there. The medical director was called about 5pm. He called the doctor to find out what the problem was. The new hire replied that there was nothing he could do as there was no conclusive evidence for treating the patient. The medical director asked him if he had been following the literature at all, the new hire said yes of course. "So what's stopping you from treating the patient", the director asked. There is no gold standard for those studies, the new doctor replied. "Does your patient care about gold standard or does she just want to be treated?" Treated. "Then go ahead and treat the patient". I need more proof. "Tell the family that. You'd be a fool to be looking for RCT gold or platinum standard as it means you're devoid of commonsense if your patient is sick and you're awaiting randomized protocols to give you proof that something works. You will never get that proof for this patient sitting or lying right in front of you at this moment, robot. Get to work and care for your patient or get out of this hospital!" I wonder how that ended for the patient.

In the midst of all the drama are the robot doctors, programmed to never think outside the box and incapable of providing creative solutions that can save a patient's life if that is what is needed. Take for example the MATH+ protocol designed by the leaders in critical care. The smart doctor would use the protocol because there is nothing else, the unwise one will say they want more proof, while letting their patients die. As I mentioned in my previous books, hyperinflammation is what kills patients in Covid-19 infection. What should be the natural response of a sensible doctor? Stopping hyperinflammation! That's exactly why the MATH+ protocol for hospitalized Covid-19 patients was a combination of **M**ethylprednisolone, High dose **A**scorbic Acid (Vitamin C), **T**hiamine and Low Molecular Weight **H**eparin as well as Zinc, melatonin, Magnesium and Famotidine. The rationale for Ascorbic acid is its antioxidant effect while thiamine helps optimize cellular oxygen use. Heparin reduces the cytokine-induced clot formation and methylprednisolone is an obvious anti-inflammatory agent. So avoid the HCQ debate if you don't want to use HCQ and treat your patients based on your knowledge of pathophysiology and pharmacology and take the fight away from ignorant journalists and the media propaganda machinery. The EVMS Protocol can be found at the EVMS website and is quite close to the MATH+ protocol.

MATH+ protocol for hospitalized Covid-19 patients:

IV **M**ethylprednisolone
- Mild hypoxia – 40mg daily until off oxygen
- Moderate – severe illness: 80mg bolus then 20mg q6h x 7 days
- Day 8: Switch to oral Prednisone and taper over 6 days

IV **A**scorbic Acid
- 3g/100ml every 6 hours x 7 days

IV **T**hiamine
- 200mg q12h x 7 days

SQ **H**eparin (LMWH)
- Stable patient on regular floor 0.5mg/kg q12h
- Critically ill or ICU patient 1mg/kg q12h (adjust for renal failure patients)
- If CrCl less than or equal to 15ml/min use unfractionated heparin.

The HCQ Debate, Caxton Opere, MD

- Monitor antifactor-Xa activity with a target range of 0.6-1.1U/ml

PLUS (+)
Zinc 75-100mg daily (ZnSO4 330mg-440mg)
Melatonin 6-12mg at night
Atorvastatin 40mg-80mg/day
Famotidine 40mg/day
Magnesium 2g IV in ICU patients

Allow permissive hypoxias tolerated without intubating until the work of breathing increases substantially. More information about the MATH protocol can be obtained from East Virginia Medical School Covid-19 Treatment website.

Remember that the patients that could not come off the ventilator after receiving toxic doses of HCQ would likely have suffered a combination of myopathy, intractable hypotension, intractable hypokalemia, and hyponatremia from the drug. Most of that dosing appears to be intentional and irresponsible.

The government protects the interests of Big Pharma not yours. Big Pharma didn't pay $233 million every year to watch a cheap drug kill their profits. WHETHER YOU ACCEPT

When you make the right conclusions from falsified evidence you will arrive at the wrong conclusions. Unnecessary deaths can only be prevented by drawing the right conclusions even from journals with distorted truths.

Clinical trials using HCQ in Hospitalized patients is oxymoronic as of May 2020. Such papers should no longer receive publication space in any worthy journal.

The Department of Defense has a Covid-19 Practice Management Guide that I had the opportunity of reading through while working with the Covid-19 Task Force Team as an independent contractor. It also contains useful information in line with the EVMS best practices.

CASIS FULL OUTPATIENT PROTOCOL FOR MILD TO MODERATE COVID-19
HCQ 400mg every 12 hours on day 1 then
HCQ 400mg daily day 2 to 5 (Total 2.4g)
Quercetin 500mg po daily x 5 days
Zinc sulfate 220mg twice daily x 5 days
Vitamin C 500mg twice daily x 5 days
Vitamin D3 2000-4000 IU daily x 5 days
Thiamine 200mg daily x 5 days
Azithromycin 500mg Day 1 and
Azithromycin 250mg daily from days 2 to 5 when indicated and safe
Aspirin 325mg once daily (if no contraindications
Incentive spirometry + cough it up and spit it out!

Sometimes patients in the ER may show drastic improvements in oxygenation within hours while awaiting an ambulance to ship them to a Covid unit in another city. Don't be surprised that by starting a treatment and adding IV Ceftriaxone 1 g with 6 or 8mg of oral Dexamethasone or 80mg of intravenous methylprednisolone, you see a drastic improvement in oxygenation.

HOSPITALIZED PATIENTS

There are multiple regimens available in hospitalized patients including the EVMS protocol, the MATH+ mentioned earlier, the DOD practice management guide. Be sure to understand the clinical status of your patient and treat accordingly. The most important elements of managing Covid-19 patients includes a pro-active approach devoid of the media and based solely on scientific thinking and not polarized policies or journals. If you think something will work and save your patient's life and perhaps livelihood, has a clear scientific rational, costs next to nothing, is relatively harmless, then I would suggest you try it as there is nothing out there that is approved for early treatment. Just be sure to operate within scientific principles and reasonable non-politicized guidelines within the scope of your practice and be the doctor conscious of your Hippocratic oath. Constantly maintain situational awareness and be ready to act emergently when patients do not seem to be showing an adequate therapeutic response to your treatment.

You can download COVID-19: REMEDIES while it is still free at www.doctorcaxton.com.

It is advisable to continue the zinc and vitamins at half the treatment dose by either taking them once daily or cutting the dose by half. If you have asthma or COPD, continue any inhaled corticosteroids. If you can, get a pulse oxymeter that tells you your oxygen saturation within seconds and always put yourself in the care of a healthcare professional or physician. The decision to add Azithromycin should be reviewed based on the likelihood of heart disease and presence of other possible infections, and an abnormal WBC. If you want to start Azithromycin, you should consider getting an EKG as well as magnesium levels as azithromycin can precipitate an arrhythmia, particularly when given to Covid-19 patients on HCQ or any other antiarrhythmic agent.

AN OPEN LABEL STUDY INTENTIONALLY DESIGNED BY BIASED SCIENTISTS TO SHOW LACK OF EFFICACY OF HCQ is inferior to observational data collected after the fact by clinicians who did not know their data would be analyzed for efficacy and were just treating patients to see what would work. I hope that's not too hard to figure out.

Rheumatololgists are the specialists with the deepest understanding of the molecules that afflict the human body. Oncologists come second in this area. Yet, I never hear epidemiologists insist that rheumatologists and oncologists be brought into the HCQ-Covid-19 conversation. Instead, it's more about how smart, how much power, how much ridicule you can extend to others, and how much of the agenda we can pursue without getting stopped. Everyone else is just a pawn, but who is Gambini, who is Cheyenko and most of all, who is George Sachs? Some of these antagonists work from home, some are surgeons whose surgery schedules have been cancelled while still getting a salary. Some own their practices or perhaps are even taking a pay cut, but the fact is they do not encounter the Covid-19 patients regularly in their protected spaces so it's an intellectual debate for them and they MUST WIN, no matter who dies.

Real scientists might consider checking Vitamin D3, zinc and ascorbate levels post-mortem in those patients that died or pre-mortem on patients hospitalized for Covid-19. But if the idea is to ensure no one has a clue about Covid-19, we'll never do such research.

A morally disempowering attack on those who have taken what they know works is one of the reasons for the greater number of deaths in the US. This is setting a dangerous precedent for future catastrophes that may guarantee wiping out the entire human race, almost.

The HCQ Debate, Caxton Opere, MD

Hearing Dr. Fauci on NBC on a replay on July 31, 2020 say that HCQ is ineffective in Covid-19 was an important catalyst to writing this book.

On Dr. Fauci's Statements and Related Media Interviews with White House Staff:
In an interview with NBC Admiral Brett Giroir, Assistant US Health Secretary and member of the Virus Task Force told NBC News

"While I respect Dr. Fauci, he is not always right. Dr Fauci is not 100 percent right and he doesn't necessarily, he admits that, have the whole national interest in mind. He looks at it from a very narrow public health point of view."

According to BBC online July 14, 2020, President Trump's economic adviser, Peter Navarra told CBS News in an interview:

"When you ask me if I listen to Dr Fauci's advice, my answer is only with caution. Dr. Fauci has been wrong on everything I have ever interacted with him on!"

"When I warned in late January in a memo of a possibly deadly pandemic, Fauci was telling the media not to worry."

"Dr. Fauci fought against Mr. Trump's courageous decision to halt flights from China, initially said the virus was low risk and flip-flopped on the use of masks."

I wonder why Dr. Fauci would fight, after all he is not an economist or politician who could be blamed for the flight ban.

Other books by the author:

COVID-19: Physician Treatment Strategies

https://www.amazon.com/dp/B07MD9D89X/ref=cm_sw_r_cp_api_i_clI0Eb8RN37KD

https://www.amazon.com/dp/B00QXQ1G4O/ref=cm_sw_r_cp_api_i_.oI0Eb2Y0T1TC

http://www.amazon.com/Female-Sexual-Arousal-Pink-Pill/dp/0970311966

http://www.amazon.com/Love-Handles-Caxton-Opere-MD/dp/0970311958

https://www.amazon.com/dp/1628575778/ref=cm_sw_r_cp_api_i_LuI0Eb5DEZV8N

MEDIA
ANGRY LATELY? Check out this video: http://youtu.be/fR2cPvxSVUc

DIVORCE DOUBLES HEART ATTACK RISK. http://youtu.be/798csRbK1jA

SOCIAL MEDIA
LinkedInwww.linkedin.com › caxton-opere-706b287
https://www.facebook.com/caxton.opere

WEB PAGE
www.doctorcaxton.com

About the Author

Caxton Opere, MD, is a board certified internist with over thirty years of clinical experience as an internist, emergency and critical care medicine physician on the frontlines of the pandemic taking care of Covid-19 patients. He is a researcher, an ordained minister, the author of multiple books on Covid-19, an excellent communicator and gifted teacher whose work on Covid-19 pandemic has been recognized by healthcare professionals around the world and by Texas Governor Greg Abbott. He is an International speaker, medical problem solver, and the pioneer of *Marriage Capital*[SM], the *5-Minute Compatibility Tests*[SM], *Divorce Medicine*[SM] and *The Medical Complications of Divorce*. He is happily married with children.